Returning to Life After the Storm

HOPE AND **WISDOM** FROM **JEWISH SOURCES**

WITH A SPECIAL MESSAGE FROM Pope Francis
FOREWORD BY Rabbi David Wolpe

Returning to Life After the Storm

HOPE AND WISDOM FROM JEWISH SOURCES

Rabbi Abraham Skorka

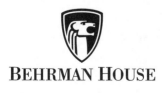

BEHRMAN HOUSE

www.behrmanhouse.com

Published by Behrman House, Inc.
Millburn, New Jersey 07041
www.behrmanhouse.com

ISBN 978-1-68115-092-5

Library of Congress Cataloging-in-Publication Data
Names: Skorka, Abraham, 1950- author.
Title: Returning to life after the storm : hope and wisdom from Jewish sources / Rabbi Abraham Skorka ; with a special message from Pope Francis ; foreword by Rabbi David Wolpe.
Description: Millburn, New Jersey : Behrman House, Inc., [2021] | Includes bibliographical references. | Summary: "As the world emerges from the COVID-19 pandemic, Jewish tradition offers a rich perspective"-- Provided by publisher.
Identifiers: LCCN 2021031579 | ISBN 9781681150925 (paperback)
Subjects: LCSH: Rabbinical literature--History and criticism. | Bible. Old Testament--History and criticism. | COVID-19 (Disease) | COVID-19 Pandemic, 2020-
Classification: LCC BM496.6 S56 2021 | DDC 296.109--dc23

LC record available at https://lccn.loc.gov/2021031579

All English translations of Hebrew scriptures are those of the author. All quotations from the Bible are referenced according to the Masoretic division of chapters and verses.

Project management by Alef Davis

Design by Zatar Creative

The publisher gratefully acknowledges Shutterstock for the following images:

INTERIOR: p. ix, xiii, 1, 3, 7, 11, 15, 19, 23, 25, 29, 33, 37, 41, 45, 51, 55, 61, 65, 69, 73, 79, 81, 83, 87, 89, 93, 97, 101, 105, 109, 111: MaraZe (wet green leaves isolated on white background, top view)

COVER: Bradley Dennien (Strong and beautiful flower growing resiliently out of crack in dark asphalt); MaraZe (wet green leaves isolated on white background, top view); photolinc (Rain drops on window glasses surface with bokeh background)

Printed in the United States of America

9 8 7 6 5 4 3 2 1

To Jana Safra, Isaac Barak, and Mila.
Grandchildren are the crown of the aged.
(Proverbs 17:6)
—A.S.

Contents

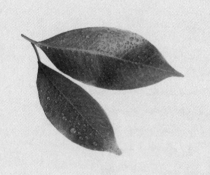

A Special Message from Pope Francis

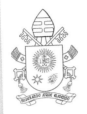

Vaticano, 5 de junio de 2021

Sr. rabino
Dr. Abraham Skorka

Querido hermano,

me alegró saber que ha compuesto un libro acerca de la pandemia en el que analiza, desde las fuentes del Judaísmo, los problemas que ha ocasionado hasta ahora.

El COVID 19 nos puso, a todos, en crisis; y de una crisis no se sale solo: o salimos todos o no salimos. Ayudar, en este tiempo, mensaje de todos los lados como respuesta a las grandes angustias producidas por este flagelo.

Estos mensajes nos ofrecerán valores para la resiliencia de una humanidad que ha sufrido y sufre tanto; y nos harán presente la verdad de que, de una crisis, no se sale igual: o salimos mejor o peores.

Deseo que su aporte inspire a muchos.

Por favor, no se olvide de rezar por mí. Lo hago por Usted.

Que el Señor le bendiga. Fraternalmente,

Francisco

The Vatican, 5 June 2021

Mr. Rabbi
Dr. Abraham Skorka

Dear brother,

I was happy to know that you have written a book about the pandemic in which you analyze, from the sources of Judaism, the problems that it has caused so far.

COVID-19 put us all in crisis; and you don't get out of a crisis alone: either we all get out or we don't get out. At this time, messages from all the creeds help in response to the great anguish produced by this scourge.

These messages will offer us values for the resilience of a humanity that has suffered and suffers so much; and they will make us aware of the truth that, from a crisis, we don't get out as we were: either we come out better or worse.

I hope your input inspires many.

Please don't forget to pray for me. I do it for you. May the Lord bless you. Fraternally,

Francisco

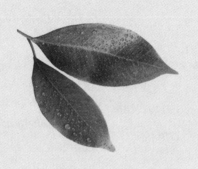

Foreword

A famous rabbinic statement declares that the Torah has seventy faces. Unfortunately, human beings have limited vision. The piece of Torah I see and value may be opaque to you, and the part that gleams in your eye I may not even see.

Especially in the modern world, riven with complexity, we need interpreters whose experience enables them to see multiple facets of our tradition. How blessed, then, to learn from Rabbi Abraham Skorka. A rabbi, a scientist, a private diplomat for the Jewish people, a man who grew up in a blessed but troubled country, a scholar with a deep understanding of other traditions, a family man, and a congregational rabbi: the range of his experience is remarkable and the fruits it yields rich and sweet. Rabbi Skorka wrings from our texts lessons about the pandemic, the Jewish future, and the fractured souls that we bear through this accelerated modern world.

Finally, Rabbi Skorka is a realist who does not fall for fashionable pessimism. Toward the closing of the book he writes that the gates of return are beginning to open. We need such a buoyant spirit to counter the fashionable despair that is both infectious and destructive. There is a blessing when one sees a wise scholar of Torah: *Shechalak Michochmato Lireav*—"Who has given of his wisdom to those who revere God." The author of this book evokes that blessing, and the book is a blessing itself.

Rabbi David Wolpe
Max Webb Senior Rabbi
Sinai Temple, Los Angeles, CA

Author's Note

I want to offer special thanks to my colleague and good friend Phillip Cunningham, with whom I have had many fruitful conversations over the last eighteen months, and to whom I am grateful for good advice and assistance in many practical matters. Dr. Cunningham is Professor of Theology and director of the Institute for Jewish-Catholic Relations at St. Joseph's University in Philadelphia. This book would not have seen the light of day without his kind help.

Introduction

We will never know if it was a human by-product or a consequence of the laws of chance that a new, highly contagious, and extremely dangerous virus emerged at the end of 2019, insinuating itself throughout the world. Its spread was subtle and quick. The fact that many world leaders minimized the gravity of the situation, motivated by political concerns, contributed to hundreds of thousands of deaths and millions of infections. On a more trivial level, people's routines were upended or curtailed entirely. Masks, social distancing, and quarantines became common as people sought to protect themselves from an epidemic that soon became a pandemic.

As days passed, uneasiness, frustration, and despair began to spread. There were many causes: the growing number of infections closer and closer to home; the loss of jobs; the disruption of the normal schooling of children and adolescents; individuals and families being forced to self-isolate; the inability to travel and to see loved ones; and much more.

Questions and doubts arose that transcended the crises of the moment. How long will it last? Am I safe? Are my loved ones safe? Why is this happening, and why now? Will everything I know and love fade away?

I am a biophysicist, a rabbi, and a Jewish educator. I have sought to understand the pandemic from all sides. Most of all, my interest in grasping our troubled present has been enhanced by my dedication to teaching the wisdom we have received from our rich Jewish past.

These chapters are written to address our questions and doubts. They were written first as an intimate diary while the pandemic was lengthening and then continued as new waves of infections, and variants of the virus, followed the initial ones. I have called the book *Returning to Life after the Storm* because I have sought insights that the emergency has produced and have tried to understand what they might mean in the long term once this nightmare is behind us.

I write to seek answers from Jewish sources for responses to our present-day problems. Judaism, in addition to asking that we follow a number of norms or mitzvot, demands that sacred texts be studied, analyzed, and interpreted in order that we better face the challenges life brings. Being religious in the Jewish tradition is not merely to repeat customs and rites handed on from generation to generation, but to creatively reinterpret them and illumine them within the principles of Judaism. This is our responsibility as Jews.

To demonstrate how important study and introspection can be, we see, for example, in the Talmud that Moses once fainted when he did not understand the teachings of Rabbi Akiva, one of the greatest sages of the Talmud—who lived fourteen hundred years after the time of Moses![1] The lesson is: the learning is never-ending!

Our Jewish daily prayers state that the Torah—a Hebrew word for what Christians often call the Pentateuch— is our life and the length of our days. In Hebrew, Torah actually means *teaching*. So, it is in the cadences of the sacred texts that Jews who fully assume their identities find the guide and inspiration for their actions.

I also believe that Jews can help those outside the Jewish community understand better how to live, and that we do this when we share our sources and the wisdom found in them. Judaism has a universal aspect that is significant for every human being. It is that part of being Jewish with which Christianity especially, and to some extent also Islam, shaped their respective creeds and spread them throughout much of the world.

We have the potential to be brothers and sisters with one another, across the differences between our respective religious traditions. As you may know, I have had this experience for many years with Pope Francis, beginning when he was the archbishop of Buenos Aires; I would listen to his sermons in the cathedral in Buenos Aires on special occasions, as a representative of the Jewish community. I told him on many occasions, then, that he uses the vocabulary of the Jewish prophets. For instance, when he would criticize national authorities on national holidays, while evaluating how the country was doing, it was in the same tone as the prophets of Israel.

In other words, it is not only Jews who learn from the Hebrew scriptures and textual tradition. And these texts are just as relevant for understanding our current situation as they are for every other time and place in the history of humankind. So, it is by delving into those overarching, universal concepts that I have written these chapters on topics of interest to me, and hopefully also to you, following a Jewish custom that comes from long ago: keep and support the memory and the meaning that we consider essential for our existence by writing testimonies about it.

What held the Jewish people together for generations and in the Diaspora were the sacred texts. The Torah, with its messages and commands, comes to life week after week with the reading and comments of the *parashah*, a weekly Torah portion that's read according to an assigned schedule on Shabbat in synagogues and in Torah study groups everywhere. Isaiah, Jeremiah, and the other prophets also come to life through the additional readings that accompany the parashah each week. We can still learn from all of them. They have much to teach us.

We have all been suffering in these days that are hopefully soon to be behind us. But one of the most important ways to be Jewish is to transcend time by means of wrestling with God through the written word. The chapters that follow seek to respond to the drama of our recent days, a drama that is still playing out around the world. We must grapple with both the problematic behaviors and the praiseworthy deeds that we have witnessed. Hopefully, we will find some insights as the human journey continues.

PART ONE

Entering the Maelstrom

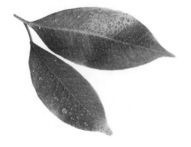

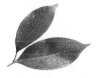

CHAPTER 1

Clothes of Arrogance, Clothes of Light

A simple virus with a decoded genetic composition has shaken all of humanity to its core. We knew who we were before this happened. We knew what we could do, what we couldn't do. We never expected that disruption of our lives on nearly every level was possible. This virus demonstrated our limitations, including the limitations of scientific knowledge when faced with novel microorganisms that pose a threat to human life.

The pandemic challenged our self-confidence, which, let's be honest, often borders on arrogance. In the early months, when the exact properties of COVID-19 were still a mystery, some people were impatient because scientists did not know enough about how the virus operates in the human body or how to treat it. We always seem to want to move fast and unimpeded. We want answers to every problem quickly. We've become spoiled. We have seen vast scientific and technological achievements over the last century, but we forget to hold a healthy awe for the earth, Creation, and an appreciation of how great our ignorance of the universe really is.

Vaccines are beginning to overcome this disease that has taken so many lives and harmed so many people. But even so, will humanity become even more arrogant? There is an arrogance in refusing the vaccine. There is also arrogance in who has access to the vaccine and who does not. And there is an arrogance in assuming that for those who have the vaccine, life will return exactly to where it was "before."

We are all thankful for advances in scientific knowledge. Our lives are often better as a result. But there can be arrogance in this, as well. Scientific research is also pursued for purposes that are not always altruistic. How often is knowledge sought for nefarious purposes to dominate others? Will the pandemic and its aftermath be used by leaders and regimes for political advantage?

The pandemic shined a bright light on the miseries caused by social inequities. The gap between the privileged and the marginalized is plain for all to see in the disparities of death, illness, and economic suffering. Those with the least resources suffer at double or triple the rate of more affluent social classes and communities. Very often, these gross disparities can be seen clearly within a single city. As I write this, similar disparities are evident from city to city, country to country, continent to continent, in access to the vaccines.

In the book of Genesis, after the first man and woman ate the fruit forbidden by God, they realized that they were naked. They sewed garments out of fig leaves to wrap around their bodies. Genesis 3:6-7 reads:

> When the woman saw that the tree was good for food and a delight to the eyes, and that the tree was desirable to make one have wisdom, she took of its fruit and ate. She also gave some to her husband, who was with

her, and he ate it. Then the eyes of both of them were opened and they knew that they were naked; and they sewed together fig leaves and made themselves loincloths.

After casting them out of Eden, "The Lord God made garments of skin for Adam and his wife and clothed them" (Gen. 3:21).

It seems that radical changes strip human beings of the protective coverings that provide them with security and shelter.

In the Midrash it is told that when the second-century sage and scribe Rabbi Meir copied a Torah scroll, he changed the letter 'ayin in the word for skin ('or) in Genesis 3:21 to the letter alef, making it into the word or, meaning "light."[2] The Midrash goes on to say that the first person's garments resembled a lantern, broad above and narrow below. But, most of all, the message that Rabbi Meir wanted to convey is that the human being, despite having sinned, received a garment of light from the Creator.[3]

A garment of light. Not a skin of shame.

What does this mean for us here and now? We must work and strive so that this light appears in all its splendor and covers us. We are each walking about with light surrounding us. Each human being must also strive to protect and defend the garment of light that is common to us all.

We have all gone through a radical change in recent months and years. Our protective coverings have been forever altered. But there is a future of light.

I wonder what clothes we will wear after the pandemic is completely over. Will we rediscover the clothing of light, or will we remain cloaked in pettiness? The pandemic caused a frenzy, stripping us of our false garments of self-assuredness, possessiveness, and arrogance. Sometimes, to our shame, we thought first or only of ourselves: our rights, our health, our families. We were afraid. We were selfish. Like our first parents in the Garden of Eden. Will we put on the same robes of arrogance and self-interest again?

I hope that, after all we have now been through, we have learned better. We will do better. We should continue to listen to Rabbi Meir and find creative and constructive ways to create and protect garments of light—for ourselves and for others.

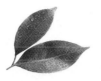

CHAPTER 2

Extravagances and Necessities

The pandemic separated extravagances from necessities. The lack of income for the many people whose jobs were lost, or who had to observe prolonged quarantines, forced us to prioritize what is really important and necessary over what are mere luxuries.

Popular culture has a way of encouraging us to imagine needs by means of subliminal advertising and subtle enticements. This is true everywhere, in every country and on every continent. I experienced it in Buenos Aires, Argentina my entire life, and I face it now where I live in Philadelphia, Pennsylvania. It isn't real. The pandemic laid all this bare. We have come to see more clearly what is truly necessary. Perhaps you are thinking of some of these necessities, even now, as you read my words.

As a result, wants that falsely became needs have now returned to their proper status in our lives. Hopefully. There are some ways in which life may never be the same again, and perhaps that's a good thing. We don't need all of that stuff.

The temptation toward human possessiveness is reflected in a very significant account in the Talmud that is set in the time of the Roman Empire. It goes like this:

Rabbi Yehudah and Rabbi Yosei and Rabbi Shimon were sitting together, and…Rabbi Yehuda began to speak, saying: How beautiful are the actions of this nation [of Rome]: they established markets, and built bridges and baths. Rabbi Yosei was silent. Rabbi Shimon bar Yochai raised his voice and said: Everything they established they did for themselves. They organized markets to seat prostitutes in them, they built baths to pamper themselves, and bridges to collect taxes.[4]

Rabbi Shimon bar Yochai, a second-century sage (to whom tradition ascribes the writing of the Zohar, the *Book of Radiance*, a sacred text of Jewish mysticism), was quite extreme in how he viewed existence. The Talmudic text goes on to assign the intemperance of his character to an overly zealous spirituality, which actually earned him a punishment from God. But in his excessively cynical opinion of Rome, there is still an unquestionable truth.

No one can deny Rome's contributions to universal culture, especially architecture, engineering, law, literature, and philosophy. From Rome came the Roman Senate; the lingua franca of the Latin language; and architectural advancements such as the impressive Colosseum, aqueducts and bridges, and roads, the likes of which were not seen again in Europe for a millennium. The Roman Empire was the glory of Western civilization. But in the eyes of the rabbis, it was spiritually very weak, even though it eventually adopted a religion that had been born from the spirituality of the Judea of which Rabbi Shimon was one of its sages.

Maimonides, the great sage and teacher of the twelfth century and one of the pillars of Jewish thought, taught that people must adopt a moderate, middle way in their behavior. Extremes are to be avoided. This is instructive for every age.

It seems to me that everything that is appealing, and beautiful, and, even in certain ways, extravagant, have their proper place in the world. We should dance and sing. Constructing great buildings is good. Paintings and sculptures, and art of all kinds are beauties to behold and expressions of the profound human spirit. May each of us be able to enjoy such things from time to time. May they not be reserved only for the few.

But when these beautiful and even extravagant things become ends in themselves—or worse, become the very center of life itself—then human life loses its ultimate meaning.[5] This is the wisdom of the sages of our Jewish tradition, and it points to why Rome was so spiritually feeble. The Romans lost sight of what was most important.

Throughout the last century, a consumerist mentality has prevailed. What is good for me, or what makes me happy, has been too central. This has driven the development and improvement of many conveniences that bring ease to our lives. Where would we be without some of the things that have been created? Consider refrigeration, microwave technology, and cellular communication, to name just a few. What our ancestors would have thought to be extravagances, we now call normal. Some of these innovations have become so common that we take them for granted.

The problem is that when we seek more and more convenience, more and more gadgets, and more and more entertainments and sources of pleasure we become like the Romans. We lose sight of what matters most. When the drive for conveniences becomes too strong in us, and in our culture, we have lost focus. Advancement and achievement too easily become ends in themselves.

With its technology and comforts, unprecedented at that time in history, Rome ruled the world. But as every child still learns in school, Rome also fell. And long before the Roman Empire came to its inglorious end, it had ignored the more important aspects of life. The vices described by Rabbi Shimon long ago were a series of corruptions upon the most precious aspect of all: our essential humanity.

I suggest that we were in a similar state before the pandemic hit. How did we measure our success, our lives? I hope that, now, our intentions are different. I hope that we have regained our sight of what matters most. May we refocus on what is most important, and of utmost necessity, as we go forward together.

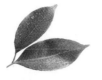

CHAPTER 3

Pandemic of Purposelessness

L ong before anyone heard of COVID-19, our communities and our cultures were afflicted by a decline of attention to the spiritual aspect of life. For good reason. After the devastation of two World Wars, the horrors of the Shoah, and the use and proliferation of atomic weapons that could eliminate our very planet, many people began to question the meaning of life, of existence itself.

Our world, it seemed, was lost. Meaning was fleeting, or at least hard to find.

There were those who looked for an answer in mysticism, for example in Kabbalah, the Jewish mystical system that arose in thirteenth-century Provence, France. This system, according to the famous scholar Gershom Scholem, formed the basis for later developments of spirituality, including the teachings of Moses ben Jacob Cordovero (1522–1570) and Isaac Luria (1534–1572).[6]

Others searching for meaning in life turned to rigid religious systems that are characterized by a strict adherence to norms and a fundamentalist stance toward traditions. This phenomenon was especially apparent in the Abrahamic religions—Judaism, Christianity, and Islam—in the late 1970s. Fundamentalisms of many kinds saw a dramatic reemergence. The most extreme of these movements propagated acts of terrorism and barbarism that spread destruction and blood to many parts of the planet.

Other people rummaged through self-help books, a New Age movement was born, and still others tried to escape their existential anguish with the use of drugs and hallucinogens to enter into alternative mental states, seeking real meaning that continued to be elusive. All of these developments signified a deep crisis of life and spirit. There was a vacuum in human life that needed filling.

At the same time, science and technology have changed human life greatly, at least in certain parts of the world. The changes have even been greater than those foreseen by futurists such as Alvin Toffler in the famous books he wrote decades ago.[7] Rapid technological changes have had a great impact on the lives of everyone and on the minds of many, and an almost religious faith in the ability of science to solve all problems has probably contributed to a further decline of belief in God and the spirit.

This, in turn, has added to people's anxiety when confronted with problems beyond the easy reach of science. So what do we do now? Without God, and without an omnipotent and omniscient science, what do we do? To whom do we turn?

The virus, and the pandemic it created, deepened and exacerbated all these trends. When people lack or do not cultivate the sense of a personal God, or any sort of spiritual aspect of life, there can be both emotional and physical consequences. I've seen this over and over in my own work, and we've witnessed this in many eras throughout history. The absence of a spiritual dimension, of a personal sense of the Transcendent, leaves people with an overwhelming loneliness.

Nothing but the Holy One can truly fill this space in our lives. The pandemic made this clearer than ever. Just as devastating as the sickness and death that it caused was the hopelessness and purposelessness it fostered in people's minds and hearts in every culture and country of the world. The answer to such a lack of hope is not to live hedonistically like Rome, or as is described in Isaiah 22:13: "Let's eat and drink because tomorrow we die." That's not the way.

There are still answers to be found in Judaism, in the God of our texts and prayers and tradition, where deep spiritual faith is not based on fundamentalist ignorance or mystical wishful thinking. As Maimonides would say, when we avoid the extremes, we find the center, and there is the truth. The God of the Bible is encountered in the dialogue of people with their own inner beings. It is rooted in being open to and discerning of the elusive and subtle presence of God. This is what we are made for.

Biblical tradition reflects this experience by portraying Abraham hearing God guiding him to another land. As it says in Genesis 12:1: "Go forth from your country, from your people and from your father's house to the land that I will show you."

Likewise, it is the "still, small voice" that moved the prophet Elijah:

> And lo, the Lord passes by. There was a great and mighty wind, splitting mountains and shattering rocks by the power of the Lord; but the Lord was not in the wind. After the wind—an earthquake; but the Lord was not in the earthquake. After the earthquake—fire; but the Lord was not in the fire. And after the fire—a thin silent voice. (1 Kgs. 19:11-12)

And it is the yearning from within that consumed the prophet Jeremiah:

> You enticed me, O Lord, and I was enticed;
> You overpowered me and You prevailed.
> I have become a laughingstock all day long,
> Everyone jeers at me.
> For every time I speak, I must cry out,
> "Lawlessness and rapine!" I shout,
> For the word of the Lord causes me
> Constant disgrace and contempt.
> I said: "I will not mention Him,
> No more will I speak His name—"
> But [His word] was like a raging fire in my heart,
> Shut up in my bones;
> I weary holding it in, but I cannot.

(Jeremiah 20:7-9)

And a sense of the nearness of the divine Presence is what enabled the psalmist to sing, "The Lord is near to all those who cry out to the Lord, to all who cry out with sincerity" (Ps. 145:18).

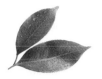

CHAPTER 4

Is Pain a Punishment?

The pandemic, like other tragedies, has prompted many people to think about the meaning of pain in human life. As has happened before in times of suffering, there are those who assume that God has sent pain—in this case, the coronavirus—as a punishment and then speculate about what might have triggered such divine wrath.

There are indeed texts in the Torah that speak of God protecting the righteous and punishing the wicked. See, for example, Deuteronomy 11:26-28:

> See, this day I set before you blessing and curse: blessing, if you obey the commandments of the Lord your God that I command upon you this day; and curse, if you do not obey the commandments of the Lord your God, but turn away from the path that I enjoin upon you this day and follow other gods, whom you have not known.[8]

There are also biblical texts that grapple with the seeming prosperity of the wicked and the suffering of the innocent righteous. For instance, this first portion of Psalm 73:

Truly is God good to Israel, to those who have a pure heart.

As for me, my feet had almost slipped, my steps were nearly led off course, for I envied the arrogant; I saw the wicked at peace.

Death has no pangs for them; their body is healthy.

They have no part in the travail of men; they are not afflicted as other men.

(Ps. 73:1-5)[9]

In other words, according to our Jewish sources, this is not a simple question with an easy answer.

The modern Hebrew term for epidemic is *mageifah*, whose root is N-G-F *(nun-gimmel-pay)*. This three-consonant pattern is found in the Bible and refers to a defeat on the battlefield or, in rabbinic texts, as a violent blow suffered.[10] Although some biblical passages attribute this suffering to the wrath of God, a rabbi such as the third-century Rabbi Yannai is remembered as insisting, "We have no comprehension of the tranquility of the wicked, nor of the suffering of the righteous."[11]

Beginning in the time when the people of Israel were tormented at the hands of the Romans, the biblical idea of God rewarding the righteous and punishing the wicked was no longer understood literally. Instead, justice was to be realized in the afterlife. Thus, we read in rabbinic literature that the payment the righteous will receive for their good deeds will be in the future to come, and the punishment of the wicked will be in hell *(Gehinnom).*[12]

After the Shoah, many rabbis and Jewish thinkers tried to make sense of the horrible deaths of millions of innocent people. This was difficult to do, although many have tried. In the end, I believe, perhaps silence is the best response. We cannot know, and perhaps we should not postulate theories.

For instance, Talmudic legend relates that God revealed to Moses the torturous fate that the greatest of the Talmudic sages, Rabbi Akiva, was going to suffer at the hands of the Romans. In this imaginative episode, Moses asks God, "Is this the reward for devotion to the Torah?" And the Creator replies, "Be silent: Be silent! This was the purpose of my thought!"[13]

So, are pain and suffering a punishment for something we have done? It is human arrogance that attributes suffering during a pandemic, or any other tragedy, to divine action. It is presumptuous for human beings to claim knowledge of the mind or activity of God.

One can argue with God or cry out to God as Job did in his pain, but one cannot expect to receive a definitive answer. Job was soothed when he felt the presence of God again.

Then there was Aaron, Moses's brother, who fell silent at the death of two of his sons (Lev. 10:3). Silence is itself a form of praise to God: "For You, silence is praise," says the psalmist (Ps. 65:2).

So, in the end, perhaps it is silence that is most meaningful for us, too, whenever we are in pain.

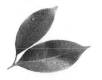

CHAPTER 5

Lessons about Leadership

The pandemic has revealed a great deal about the nature of leadership—what works, what doesn't. In its glare, we have been able to readily distinguish leaders who are motivated to serve and bring out the best qualities of their people, from those whose policies seem driven only by the ambition for power. In some nations, the people themselves elected leaders who, in times of crisis, bring out the worst, or reveal the worst, in us.

Why would we choose such leaders?

After the Second World War, this question was analyzed by many different thinkers, such as Erich Fromm in his book *The Fear of Freedom*. Fromm reflected:

> We have been compelled to recognize that millions in Germany were as eager to surrender their freedom as their fathers were to fight for it; that instead of wanting freedom, they sought for ways to escape from it; that other millions were indifferent and did not believe the defence of freedom to be worth fighting and dying for.[14]

But these are, in fact, ancient questions, already found in the biblical book of Judges through the story of Gideon.

The Bible describes Gideon's rejection of the people's proposal that he become their king, responding that God is the only true monarch (Judg. 8:22-23). The people wanted to relinquish their freedom. They said to Gideon: "Rule over us, you, your son, and then your grandson." But Gideon replied, "I will not...only the Lord God will rule over you."

Further on, we read about the insatiable ambition of Abimelech, Gideon's son, who killed seventy of his half-brothers in order to acquire power. Still later, we find the parable of Jotham (Judg. 9:8-15), which teaches that people who are productive and fruitful do not crave power, leaving a vacuum that destructive leaders tend to fill.

These biblical passages depict the entire spectrum of leadership, from the greatness of those who lead in service for the good of others to those infected by what in ancient Greece was known as hubris: arrogant self-confidence and self-adoration. We've known too many such leaders, especially in recent times.

Could this current crisis, with all its devastation, leading to many shattered lives and damaged communities, serve to remove selfishness, self-centeredness, and egotism from the minds and hearts of our leaders? Is it possible that a new leadership of service might reemerge when we come fully out of this disruptive storm?

The twentieth century has witnessed the rise of too many evil leaders. Selfish. Arrogant. Mad? Figures such as Mussolini, Hitler, Stalin, Pol Pot, and Idi Amin knew how to draw a large portion of their people to follow them, by inspiring their worst instincts, and wreaking chaos and devastation. They often saw themselves as new Caesars who were destined to conquer the world and create new empires. The Roman, Carolingian, and Napoleonic Empires served as their models and ideals.

In the twenty-first century, there are now new channels of domination. For instance, there are international corporations that possess much greater economic power than many nations or even groups of nations do. Their power is frightening in the same manner that a fascist regime once was. Today's vast empires are often built on the basis of technological supremacy rather than by military conquest. Likewise, wars have become technological, reaching high degrees of sophistication, and those who win are those who have what others have not. Hunger, misery, and fanaticism continue to multiply in the midst of this new reality in which the cumulative knowledge now available to combat all our ills is not always used for the good of all.

Does it take a pandemic to induce world leaders to turn their hearts to the service of their people rather than their domination? Will we begin to again see it as our responsibility to care for the people of all nations and not only for ourselves? I hope that we will again value freedom and elect leaders who seek to free the bonds of all people, by every means at their disposal. I also wonder if we will finally now see the even bigger problem with our attitudes of domination: the need to care for the planet we all share. Our problems are much larger than what one country can accomplish on its own.

The rabbis of the Talmud knew the push and the pull in every human heart between self-interest and interest in the community at large. They said:

If I am not for myself, who will be for me?

If I am for myself only, what am I?

If not now—when?[15]

21

This reflects again the both/and truth from Maimonides.[16] We can care for ourselves and also care for others. We care for ourselves, in fact, *by caring for others.*

My hope is that this novel virus will shock our leaders out of their self-interest. And if only we would no longer elect leaders who appeal to our most selfish interests! May this crisis prompt us to look to a new kind of leader, one who possesses qualities that reflect the best qualities in us.

PART TWO

Inside the Storm

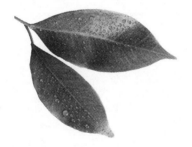

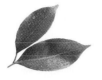

CHAPTER 6

Resilience and Remembrance

There are two challenges that the current plague places before us. On the one hand, there is a need for resilience in the face of economic, psychological, and emotional collapse and—in too many cases—the loss of loved ones. On the other hand, we must ask ourselves what lessons we can learn from such dire experiences.

People have a way of overcoming or circumventing obstacles as they pursue paths of recovery and resilience. But when it comes to the challenge of discerning what lessons we can learn, questions arise: How will we make meaning out of these days of difficulty? Will we be able to forget what needs forgetting and remember the lessons we should retain for the future? Will our memories be fragile, will we simply seek to avoid pain? Will those who were less affected by the pandemic only remember it as an annoying time and be insensitive to the suffering of others?

Memory is an essential theme in the Bible. Moses, in his "farewell address" to the people, cries out, saying: "Remember the days of old, consider the generations of ages past. Ask your father and he will tell you, your elders and they will say to you" (Deut. 32:7). Similarly, the sanctity of Shabbat is to be remembered every seven days (Exod. 20:7-10 or 20:8-11 according to another tradition), and the day of becoming free after leaving the land of Egypt should be recalled every day that people live (Deut. 16:3).

We are to be a remembering people. Psalm 90:12 says: "Teach us to count our days rightly, that we may obtain a wise heart."

We are not made to endure high levels of pain, frustration, and discomfort for long periods of time. Life soon begins to feel unbearable. Human resilience involves distancing ourselves from heartbreaking moments of pain in order to cope with them. Nonetheless, traumas have a significance that should forever live in, and guide, our memories. If what happened to us is erased, avoided, or forgotten, the acquired experience, which can help us face life and pass lessons on to our children, vanishes as well.

This is why memory occupies such a central place in the Jewish tradition. Memory transforms people into families and families into peoples and nations. It is also the framework that supports the values of the individual and of society. When memory is erased, we may maintain a common language, idioms, and traditions, but our values will have become a blank slate. This explains both the conformity of people who are enthralled and indoctrinated by demagogues, and the actions of those who cunningly manipulate others for their own purposes. Without memory, societies are transformed into mobs and people into zombies.

The Jewish people, despite having lost sovereignty over the land of Israel, never forgot the pain of its destruction at the hands of the Romans. Eleven centuries after the destruction of Jerusalem, Maimonides codified in the *Mishneh Torah*, based on the teachings of the Talmudic Sages, the symbols we have to follow in order to remember the Temple:

Since the Temple was destroyed, the Sages of that generation ordained that one should never build a building that is whitewashed and ornamented like the building of kings. Instead, one plasters his house with plaster and whitewashes it with lime and leaves over without lime a space an ell by an ell, opposite from the entrance....[17]

They also ordained that one who sets a table to make a meal for guests should leave an empty place; and when a woman has a set of jewelry made for her from silver and gold, she should leave off one of the pieces of jewelry to which she is accustomed, so that the jewelry is incomplete; and when a groom marries a woman, he should take burnt ashes and put it on his head in the place of where the tefillin would normally lay. All of these things are so as to remember Jerusalem, as it is stated: "If I forget you, O Jerusalem, let my right hand wither. Let my tongue stick to my palate if I do not remember you, if I do not raise up Jerusalem above my greatest joy" (Ps. 137:5-6).

Although the traditions have changed over time (for instance, the groom breaks a glass under the wedding canopy in place of putting burnt ashes on his forehead), their purpose remains the same: to recall the pain of destruction. We are to remember, and to put that memory to use in our lives. The periods of pain and suffering are not supposed to paralyze and impede us but lead us to positive action.

We Jews have learned to do this, due to much practice. For example, after more than two thousand years in which our original language, Hebrew, was used only for liturgical purposes, it was transformed by modern Jews into a living language on their way back to their ancestral land. Similar resilience was shown after the atrocities of the Crusades, the Spanish Inquisition, the pogroms of the early modern period, and the singular Shoah. After each of these tragedies there was a process of elaborating the sufferings and pain, together with teaching the memory of what happened. "Memory is the lifeblood of a Jewish being," says Rabbi Ismar Schorsch, the Chancellor Emeritus of The Jewish Theological Seminary, who was himself born in Nazi Germany.[18]

In our day, too, as we emerge from this pandemic, it is imperative for us to busy ourselves with resilience and remembrance. They complement each other in a healthy human life.

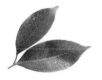

CHAPTER 7

An Ethic for Everyone

The book of Genesis, which is core to all three of the Abrahamic religions, tells us that the wrath of God was provoked by the widespread sinning of human beings:

> The Lord saw how great was man's wickedness on earth and how every thought devised by his mind was only evil all the time. And the Lord regretted that He had made man on earth, and His heart was saddened....The earth was corrupt before God; the earth was filled with lawlessness. When God saw how corrupt the earth was, for all flesh had corrupted its ways upon the earth, God said to Noah...(Gen. 6:5-6, 11-12)

The Almighty, through a huge flood, then destroys every living being except for one human family, that of Noah, and the animals that were preserved in his ark.

Genesis narrates that once the Flood ceased, the survivors had to face a devastated world. They had to begin humanity anew. God made a pact with them. God gave human beings a code of ethics, different from the original one given to Adam, who, for example, was only allowed to eat vegetables (Gen.

1:29). From now on, human beings were allowed to eat animals (Gen. 9:3).[19]

Another interesting element also appears in this new covenant of God with the human remnant. God promises never to send another massive flood upon the earth. To the family traumatized by the devastation, God gives the reassurance they need to face the future. Noah, whose name can mean "consoler" or "comforter" (Gen. 5:29), and his family even behold a rainbow in the sky as a sign of God's covenantal promise:

> God further said. "This is the sign of the covenant that I am establishing between Me and you, and every living creature with you, for all ages to come. I have set My bow in the clouds, and it shall be as a sign of the covenant between Me and the earth." (Gen. 9:12-13).

God, as it were, hangs up the weapon of the bow in the sky, never again to take it up against his own creation.

This story may subtly suggest that if the world is to be destroyed in some future time, it will be by the deeds of humanity and not by an act of God.

Rabbinic tradition understood that God's pact with Noah included seven precepts that all of Noah's descendants were expected to observe. These were prohibitions against murder, blasphemy, idolatry, theft, sexual immorality, eating a living animal, and the need to establish a system of justice. The rabbis saw these rules as the basic norms for all civilized people.[20]

According to the Talmud, non-Jews, people who are not part of the Torah Covenant from Mount Sinai,[21] must also follow these seven precepts in order to be considered righteous, or good people, by Jewish standards. Later, in the Middle Ages, Maimonides taught, "Anyone who [is not a Jew and] accepts the seven [Noahide] precepts and is careful to fulfill them is considered one of the pious among the peoples and has a share in the World to Come."[22] We see in this tradition of the Noahide laws an effort to apply basic behavioral standards to all of humanity.

A similar impulse toward a universal ethic is evident among other people as well. For instance, in the Roman Empire, the concept of the *jus gentium*, or "law of nations," developed as a set of customs with which all nations should comply regardless of their particular or national civil laws. This was related to *jus naturale*, or "natural law," which, according to the second-century Roman legal expert Gaius were laws that "natural reason has established among all peoples."[23] Combined with the thinking of several Greek philosophers, especially Aristotle, this notion of natural law would eventually become a key concept in Christianity, as norms built into the fabric of human life by God, which all people could discover.

There are some resonances between Christian thinking about natural law and the Jewish Noahide commandments. In fact, in 1640, the English jurist John Selden, in his *De jure Naturali et gentium juxta disciplinam Ebraeroum (On the Law of Nature and Nations Compared with Hebrew Teaching)*, argued that natural law was based upon the Noahide laws.

Whatever one thinks of such Jewish, Christian, or secular attempts to compose universal norms for everyone, the impulse to do so seems widespread. We need to have, and live by, certain universal laws or norms that guide the behavior of good people.

The COVID-19 pandemic raised questions about universal access to health care, to vaccines, and to the necessities of life that brought to the forefront concern for a worldwide ethical code—minimum standards to which all people and nations should deeply commit themselves. The 1948 United Nations' "Universal Declaration of Human Rights" was an important step in this direction, but it is frequently paid only lip service and not effectively implemented.

Here again, religious perceptions may be helpful. Ecclesiastes 7:13 states, "Consider God's work! Who can straighten what God has twisted?" The rabbinic midrash Kohelet Rabbah comments on this, saying:

> When the Holy One, blessed be He, created the first human being, He took him and led him around all the trees of the Garden of Eden and said: "Look at My works, how beautiful and praiseworthy they are! And everything I have created, it was for you that I created it all. Be careful not to corrupt and destroy My world: if you corrupt it, there is no one to repair it after you."[24]

May we all pay attention to this insight. It is ancient—yet more relevant and necessary than ever before. The future of our children and grandchildren and generations to come is at stake if humanity fails to compose and embrace common ethics for everyone.

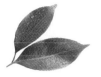

CHAPTER 8

To Tend It and Keep It

Some large cities proved to be particularly vulnerable in the early days of the spread of COVID-19. The great human conglomerates, the concrete jungles that house millions of human beings, are centers of creativity and culture but throughout history have also provided environments for the rapid dissemination of diseases. Indeed, there is a possibility that the very origins of the pandemic are the result of an overcrowding of people and animals in unsanitary marketplaces.

The Bible generally takes a dim view of cities. It describes Cain, the one who was doomed to wander in punishment for murdering his brother, as the builder of the first city for his son and his descendants (Gen. 4:17). This probably reflects the ancient development of agriculture that could support an urban culture. According to the biblical account, Noah turned to viticulture after the Flood ended (Gen. 9:20), and his descendant Nimrod built major cities (Gen. 10:9-11). The sages of the Talmud then considered Nimrod the main force behind the effort to build the Tower of Babel,[25] using technology that had developed in his time to goad his people "to make a name for [them]selves" (Gen. 11:3-4), thereby rebelling against God.

There is a midrash (it is a late text from the eighth or ninth century) that illustrates the sin of the builders of the Tower of Babel. It says that when in the process of construction a brick was accidentally lost, everyone lamented. But when a man died, nobody cared.[26] Today, we might say that the story shows the dangers of valuing our technological prowess more than human life.

Alternatively, these biblical and Talmudic perspectives could also be seen as warning against the danger of separating ourselves from the natural world by withdrawing inside artificial bubbles of our own making. Moreover, the raw materials we use to build our cities and power our technologies often degrade or destroy the environment itself.

Isn't it interesting how the Book of Exodus specifies that the seven-branched menorahs (lampstands) were to have fruits and flowers carved on them (Exod. 25:31-40)? Two of those verses detailing the instructions God gives to the Israelites, for instance, has God telling them:

> Six branches shall come out from its sides, three branches from one side of the lampstand and three branches from the other side of the lampstand. On one branch there shall be three cups shaped like almond-blossoms, each with calyx and petals, and there shall be three cups shaped like almond-blossoms on the next branch, each with calyx and petals; so for all six branches that proceed out from the lampstand (Exod. 25: 32-33).

Similarly, the Temple in Jerusalem, built atop a mountain surrounded by the city, was required to be adorned with decorative images of living nature, and the stones on its walls had to be covered with wood of different species (see 1 Kings 6). The liturgical festivals also were timed in accordance with the rhythms of nature. Surely the objective of all these practices was to remind everyone entering a sacred space of the human dependence on the Land of Israel and therefore of the need to care for it.

Such wisdom is ancient, biblical, and Jewish, but it needn't be any of those things to be important—it is also simply common sense.

The spiritual deformation that can result from the concentration of human beings in tiny areas is the basis for the criticisms of the influential thinker José Ortega y Gasset, who rejected despotic movements in Europe in the first half of the twentieth century. Ortega y Gasset recognized population overcrowding as a symptom leading to greater problems. He called it "the fact of agglomeration." He said: "Towns are full of people, houses full of tenants, hotels full of guests, trains full of travelers, cafes full of customers, parks full of promenaders, consulting-rooms of famous doctors full of patients, theatres full of spectators, and beaches full of bathers." And, "What previously was, in general, no problem, now begins to be an everyday one, namely, to find room."[27] So there are many reasons to have a dim view of cities, and a Spanish philosopher provides some as well.

Simply put, we need more than cities. *Adamah* is the Hebrew word used in the Creation account of Genesis 2 to mean the "ground" or "soil" that the first human being is required by God to caretake. And the name of the first human being, Adam, is of the same root. We should remember our essential relationship with the ground we walk upon and to which we are intimately linked.

The lack of direct contact with nature that characterizes the lives of inhabitants of our great cement forests prompted the Catalan architect, Antoní Gaudí, to create new architectural forms to connect human beings with the natural world. Many have learned from him since then, and city planners focus on this good work frequently today. We sometimes say that this makes our cities more "livable"—which is the most basic way to put it!

Perhaps the quarantines and isolation caused by the current pandemic will remind us that we are not above life, but we are a part of the one and only web of life. We are not to live "above" the earth, as its dominators, but we have been made responsible by the Creator "to tend it and keep it" (Gen. 2:15).

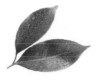

CHAPTER 9

A Signal of New Possibilities

Many have linked the pandemic to the plagues narrated in the Book of Exodus. God sent those plagues against the Egyptian pharaoh and his people to compel the liberation of the enslaved children of Israel. However, in making this connection, there is danger that a dogmatic or strained reading of the text could lead to some exaggerated conclusions.

You have probably heard or read the sort of exaggerated conclusions to which I am alluding. There are those who preach that the pandemic was a punishment of God upon humanity, or even worse, there are those who point to some specific sin or sins and say, "See, surely that is what caused this to happen to us. Repent!"

We need to better understand what it means to experience a sign or a signal from the Lord God.

Two relevant verses are found in Exodus 10:1-2:

Then the Lord said to Moses: Go to Pharaoh, for I have hardened his heart and the heart of his servants in order that I may perform these *signs* of mine among them and that you may recount in the ears of your son and grandson how I made a fool of the Egyptians and what *signs* I did among them, so that you may know that I am the Lord.

The Hebrew word *ot* for "sign" has two connotations in the Bible. On the one hand, it refers to an indication or signal of a message that must be remembered, such as the sign that God placed upon Cain for his protection (see Genesis 4:15), or the rainbow that marks the covenant God made with Noah and his family (Gen. 9:11-16). On the other hand, it may be a special sign connoting a supernatural or miraculous event, as is mentioned in Deuteronomy 13:2 or Deuteronomy 26:8: "The Lord brought us forth out of Egypt by a mighty hand, by an outstretched arm and awesome power, and by signs and portents."

In Exodus 10, the term can also be understood to refer to both a message that should never be forgotten as well as supernatural acts. The plagues appeared miraculously. They should be remembered as a judgment upon the powerless pagan deities in which the Egyptians believed (Exod. 12:12).

So, was the pandemic a divine sign? I don't think so. If it was a sign of anything, it was a reminder that we are arrogant people—like Pharoah, perhaps—who in many ways brought this pestilence, particularly in many of its complications and mishandlings, upon ourselves.

Additionally, in Exodus 10:2, God prescribes that the people of Israel should tell their children and their children's children about the signs that God performed in Egypt. Thus, they will know that the God of Israel is the almighty Lord of all existence. Even more, the freedom that the plagues brought about prepared the Hebrews to receive the Torah at Mount Sinai. It was God's gift of the Torah to Israel that revealed a new way of living that was inconceivable to the Hebrews as long as they were enslaved. They had to become open to a new situation. This was a landmark moment in history that the children of Israel should celebrate forever.

Does the coronavirus pandemic send a similar message to us today?

One might first ask whether this pandemic will also mark a milestone in human history. Surely the answer is yes. The economic and social disasters produced by the disease, the millions of deaths worldwide, and the upheavals in daily life everywhere on the globe will remain embedded not only in our memories but in our lives and the lives of our children and grandchildren for generations.

The more interesting question is whether this watershed moment will prompt us to imagine new ways of thinking and living. Will religious people become more open to the more human-serving and less dogmatic spiritualities advocated in the last century by Martin Buber, Abraham Joshua Heschel, and André Neher?[28] Will today's experience of shared suffering on a global scale chasten us and make us newly appreciate the transcendent value of human life? Will the travails of our time help us develop a more mature vision of God, one that understands that a relationship of deep dialogue between humanity and God and among all branches of the human family is the way forward?

These are the real questions to be asked. In the case of the plagues of Egypt, the Torah reveals explicitly that they were sent by God, otherwise it is forbidden to assert that some of the bad things that affect human beings were sent by Him to punish them for their misbehaviors. As we read in the Talmud:

If torments are afflicting a person, if illnesses are afflicting him, or if he is burying his children, one may not say to him in the manner that the friends of Job said to him: "Is not your fear of God your confidence, and your hope the integrity of your ways? Remember, please, who being innocent ever perished? " (Job 4:6–7)[29]

In other words, certainly you sinned, otherwise you would not have suffered misfortune.

So before we make assertions on behalf of God, pointing to signs and signals of divine activity, we should take a close, introspective look at our own failures.

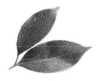

CHAPTER 10

The Days of Awe

Ritual prayers in Judaism, with a few rare exceptions, are composed in the plural. We bring our own feelings to the act of prayer, but offering them to God is most often done in community. This is why Jewish tradition so highly values communal prayer over prayers said in private.[30] Only when people are gathered together are prayers offered in their fullness.

During the first pandemic year, unlike any other time in human memory, the assembling of Jews in synagogues to mark the start of a new year was limited and constrained. Necessary protocols of social distancing, demanded by the pandemic, made it nearly impossible to make the High Holy Days of Awe meaningful. We couldn't be together. Gathering with others, joining together in singing, echoing the same prayers side-by-side, and sharing common feelings at this most important time of the year were curtailed, and in some instances, cancelled. The companionship we are so accustomed to finding in each other had to be found more in the mind and heart since physical closeness was absent.

The Days of Awe *(Yamim Nora'im)*, including Rosh Hashanah (the New Year) and Yom Kippur (the Day of Atonement), are the time when God judges all humanity, both individually and as peoples. It is a time for a critical self-analysis of our lives and existence. Who am I? Who am I in relationship to God? Who are we?

This self-review is called *cheshbon hanefesh*, a reckoning of one's being, which is similar to what Catholics call an "examination of conscience." This self-examination, of course, is about much more than ourselves—it concerns our relationship with others as well. The distancing compelled by the virus required us to conduct a deeper inward search as we examined our behaviors toward others. In most instances, we were unable even to greet each other, let alone reconcile with one another, when personal reconciliation is what a proper reckoning calls for.

But it is always good to consider the positive side of any situation, no matter how dire it may seem. Despite the unprecedented Days of Awe we had to undergo, it occurred to me then that I was suddenly better able to sit with myself and pray. I was better able to listen to the voice inside me that helped direct my reckoning—my self-examination—and it was a wonderful experience to do this.

Prayers that cannot be offered in community can lead an individual Jew to spend more time in introspective reflection. Perhaps this will enable each of us to draw closer to how God sees us in the days of divine judgment now and in the future.

We cry out to the Creator in our prayers to help us be unified in knowing how to act with a full heart according to God's will. One of the most eloquent prayers begins with the cry: "Hear our voices, Lord our God, have mercy and compassion on us!" Then follow words from Psalms 51:13 and 71:9, which in the Bible are presented as personal pleas of King David but are rephrased in the plural in the prayer book:

Do not cast us out of Your presence or take Your Holy
Spirit away from us.

Do not cast us off in old age; when our strength fails,
do not forsake us!

In the book of Psalms, these are utterances that express
a person's most particular and intimate desires. However, in
the synagogue, the individual prayer acquires a superlative
significance when, starting from an individual, it extends to
embrace others in the whole community and, ultimately, all of
humanity.

The pandemic will continue to afflict us with uncertainty,
and even fear, pain, and anguish. But it has also joined individuals and nations together with common concerns. We were not
exactly praying communally as we worked to solve the myriad
problems associated with overcoming the deadly virus among
us, but we did often learn new and better ways to communicate
across communities, nations, and religious divides.

We need to remember those ways of cooperation and working
together.

Going forward, I hope there will be discerning people who
see these developments as a sign of our need for more unity that
values differences, overcoming the ways that differences turn
into insurmountable barriers. Will this perception contribute
to that universal unity that God intends so that all people will
do justice, love kindness, and walk humbly with their Creator
(Mic. 6:8)? Will widespread and sincere dialogue be achieved in
which each of us is able to maintain our identity while feeling
ennobled to experience others in all their distinctiveness?

At the beginning of each New Year, during the Days of Awe,
we Jews ask God to judge humanity with mercy and benevo-
lence. We are bold to ask, while feeling the presence of others,

even in a time of social distancing. The pandemic was only one of the many increasingly complex threats that are challenging a world that is rapidly growing in human numbers and needs. Like the prayers of the Days of Awe, these challenges compel us to understand that we all share the same situation in this earthly reality and that the destiny of each of us is inextricably linked to that of everyone else.

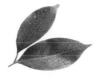

CHAPTER 11

Reflections on an Unusual Yom Kippur

As I mentioned in the last chapter, the *t'filot,* or prayers, of the Days of Awe were a particular challenge during the pandemic year. Everything was different and strange. It was a struggle to feel the spirit of Rosh Hashanah and Yom Kippur while kept apart from one another.

Being isolated meant that our communal spirituality had to be invoked from our memories of the past. As I said in *On Heaven and Earth,* the book of conversations composed with Jorge Mario Bergoglio, now Pope Francis:

> The worst thing that can happen to our relationship with God is not that we fight with Him but that we become indifferent. A religious man, even in the worst of times, will continue talking to God, just as thousands of people did when they went into the gas chambers to die, shouting, "Hear O Israel, The Lord is God, The Lord is One!" which is our declaration of faith. Despite everything, they continued believing in Him. For our Yom Kippur (Day

of Atonement) prayer service, we have incorporated a story about a document that was found in the ruins of the Warsaw Ghetto, in which the author relates that his wife and sons had died and that he is the only member of his family to have survived. He addresses God with a great deal of pain, yet there comes a part when he says that however much he is put to the test, he will continue to believe in Him. That is true faith.[31]

The pandemic also forced us to take seriously the insight of Rabbi Eliezer that "if someone makes his prayers mechanical, it is not [really] supplication."[32] There is no deep intention, no exercise of the will and heart.

The Talmud relates that when Rabbi Yishma'el ben Elisha, as high priest, entered the Holy of Holies on a certain Yom Kippur, he saw a vision of God who said to him:

> "Yishma'el, my son, bless Me!" [Yishma'el said:] May it be Your will that Your mercy overcome Your anger, and may Your mercy prevail over Your other attributes, and may You act toward Your children with the attribute of mercy, and may You enter before them beyond the letter of the law." The Holy One, Blessed be He, nodded and accepted the blessing.

What does this mean? The Talmud imagines that we should not take the blessing of an ordinary person lightly.[33] If God asked for and accepted someone's blessing, all the more so should we value the blessings of others. We must consciously pursue stronger relationships with those separated from us.

Any Yom Kippur we may find many moments of solitude, such as the one felt by that high priest when he entered the Holy of Holies. Especially on such an extraordinary day, we should feel as never before a sense of responsibility, as that priest did, for all of our people and for all people everywhere. An obligation toward others lies in the hands of all Jews, no matter their spiritual experiences or official responsibilities, no matter the vastness or smallness of their potential contributions. This responsibility toward others is always fundamental.

In his time, Moses obtained God's forgiveness for the people of Israel for worshiping the golden calf (Num. 14:20). So, too, Rabbi Yishma'el received God's mercy for the people by uttering his blessing. When praying, people should see themselves as offering something very humble but also transcendent and unique. We ought not to compare ourselves to Moses or to Rabbi Yishma'el, but we should feel that the continuation of their legacy depends on the authenticity and sincerity of our own prayers. As Rabbi Zusya of Hanipoli (died 1800) taught: "In the coming world, they will not ask me: 'Why were you not Moses?' They will ask me: 'Why were you not Zusya?'"[34]

By disrupting our community practices, the pandemic forced us, on the one hand, to interact via telephone, Zoom, and many other means of communication, and, on the other hand, to redefine the way in which we pray, study Torah, and express our affections and emotions.

Each year, as the Days of Awe arrive, images of our grandparents, parents, and teachers emerge from our memories, causing us to celebrate these moments with real feeling. In the *Yamim Nora'im* of years subsequent to the pandemic, we will also call to mind our memories of when we could not hug and embrace each other.

Memory should be an inspiring force to renew our prayers. Its power is masterfully revealed in a story told by Rabbi Yisra'el of Ruzhin, who said:

Once the holy Ba'al Shem Tov wanted to save the life of a sick boy for whom he had a lot of affection. He ordered a candle of pure wax to be brought to him, took it to the forest, secured it to a tree, and lit it. Then he delivered a long prayer. The candle burned all night. By morning, the boy was fine.

When my great-grandfather, the Great Maggid [Dov Ber of Mezeritch], who was a disciple of the holy Ba'al Shem Tov, wanted to achieve a similar cure, he no longer knew the secret meaning of the words he had to focus on. He did what his teacher had done and invoked his name. And his efforts were successful.

When Rabbi Mosheh Leib of Sassov, the disciple of the Great Maggid's disciple, wanted to achieve such a cure, he said: "We no longer even have the power to do what was done. But I'll tell the story of how it happened, and God will help." And his efforts were successful. [35]

Finally, the two complementary readings to the Yom Kippur Torah readings—the *haftarot*—have in common the cry of a prophet for the revitalization of our attitudes. (Isa. 57:14-58:14) cries out to the people for a sincere fast during which the bonds of iniquity are undone, and social justice and solidarity are reestablished as the values that shape our conduct. Not a mere meeting in the Temple, nor a formal fast, the prophet calls on the people to change their attitude toward others in order to reexperience Yom Kippur. On a universal scale, we find the same message in the text of Jonah: the inhabitants of Nineveh kept a fast in which they made a transformative decision: to forsake all immorality. It was a turning point in their lives; their prayer was not a mere recitation.

The pandemic prevented us from repeating patterns and deprived us of moments that had become habits learned over generations. Perhaps it was a divine design to create a different fast so that we would better understand the message of Isaiah and Jonah and respond to the prophetic voice in our midst with deeper commitment.

Uncertainty necessarily characterizes the day of divine judgment and our requests for forgiveness. We've been thoroughly reminded of uncertainty in these recent days. After so many spectacular advances in science and technology, many medical problems seemed curable. Only the unresolved challenges of the past, such as cancer, remained, concerning which much progress has been made. But the coronavirus reminded us of our limitations. Our weaknesses resurfaced, and they distressed us. They added a poignant dimension to the questions that the *t'filah* invites us to ask ourselves each morning: What is our life? What is our prayer? What is our righteousness before You, O God?

In the *piyut* (liturgical poem) *Unetaneh Tokef*, it is said that in Heaven during the Days of Awe, God determines who is to live and who is to die. Who in his time and who before his time? Who in the earthquake and who in the pandemic? We tremble before these questions and the uncertainty of the Holy One's decision. We cannot—we will not ever—understand them fully.

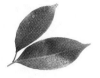

CHAPTER 12

The Blessing of Bewilderment

As you read this (or, at least, as this book goes to press), the pandemic began about two years ago. Vaccines have since been created and have been found mostly effective, but too many people have also refused to take them, and too many people in the world have not had easy access to them. Conclusive solutions to the overall problem facing us are not yet fully in sight.

To further complicate things, for some individuals, the disease has only seemed to manifest itself in a very mild form, while in others, it has unpredictably and devastatingly attacked various parts of the body. Millions of people have recovered without much difficulty, but millions of others have died, sometimes rapidly. There are still unknown factors that play an important role in the behavior of this virus, making it more difficult to find effective vaccines for the long haul and treatments for all.

Perhaps science today finds itself in a similar position as it was at the beginning of the twentieth century, when the so-called Spanish flu was raging. Many people, scientists included, thought that most of the secrets of nature had already been—or were about to be—discovered. They felt that only a few residual details remained to be resolved. For them, the 1918 influenza pandemic was an uncomfortable eye-opener.

This brings to mind an article I published in *La Nación* in the year 2000 to mark the one-hundredth anniversary of physicist Max Planck's groundbreaking work in quantum mechanics. I wrote that, on December 14, 1900, Planck announced that his calculations made it clear that energy is not absorbed or emitted continuously by bodies but in strictly defined quantities called "quanta."

This was important because it was science's first great step in delving into the essence of the fundamental constituents of matter. It was the beginning of a new paradigm in physics. From the days of Isaac Newton (1643-1727) until the beginning of the twentieth century, physics successfully explained many natural phenomena through mechanistic models, such as using mathematical formulas to calculate the motions of the planets. Every object seemed susceptible to analysis on the basis of its position, speed, and energy. Nature itself appeared to be like a great machine whose operations could be encapsulated in mathematical equations. However, Planck's research called all that into question. This was expressed by Plank's colleague Werner Heisenberg in 1927 in his famous uncertainty principle, which stated that it is impossible to speak confidently of the position of subatomic particles, but only of the probability that they are at a certain point or of the likelihood that they will follow a particular path. This quantum theory triggered a continuing debate about whether physical reality is ultimately intentionally caused or is purely random.

As I wrote then, perplexity and amazement had (thankfully) returned to science. You don't have to be a theologian or a rabbi to say this. I'm saying it also as a scientist. We need humility in the face of our research and advancements.

As physicist Niels Bohr put it in 1952, "If there are those who do not feel deeply surprised when they first come into contact with quantum theory, the only explanation is that they have not understood it." Bewilderment and wonder make us aware of the limits of our knowledge but also encourage us to continue searching for fuller understandings.

To return to the world of the pandemic, it seems that we have again been in a period that calls upon us to recognize our limitations and our lack of total control over the world. Perplexity and doubt are not restricted to science. All philosophical systems and religious traditions must respond to the wonder of existence.

We didn't need the pandemic to teach us this. The overwhelming evidence of climate change due to human factors has yet to convince us that we aren't here to dominate the planet. Nor do we control it. Now, the pandemic has reinforced this teaching for us. Will we listen? Will we hear it? This is "teaching," or Torah, too.

We seem unable to listen. One common response is to resort to fanaticism and fundamentalism, establishing rigid absolutes in a futile effort to cover over our limits and doubts. Everything is thought to be perfectly defined, so there is no room for doubt or any need to search further. It is not surprising that tyrants and dictators have banned the teaching of modern mathematics and other sciences, claiming that they "disturb the mind."[36]

Perplexity also challenges the widespread expectation in Western culture of quick resolutions to puzzles and problems. The unanswered question is abhorred. Even though quantum research reveals glaring uncertainties, people often think of science as a source of omniscience. Yet science itself teaches us that a question without an immediate answer is extremely valuable because it prompts the development of new theories that can be tested and new research that can be pursued.

These thoughts resonate with my Jewish faith. Although God is revealed to humanity in the Bible, God remains a mystery because human minds are unable to fathom God's magnificence. This causes them to continue inquiring and seeking the presence of a higher power. Abraham, surely, was perplexed by the great challenges that God placed before him, yet in his struggle to cope with them, he found new dimensions of faith. Moses was confounded by being asked to speak on behalf of God because he was ineloquent and slow of speech. Job was bewildered by his undeserved suffering but eventually became contented. The Bible seems to teach us that faith is born when an awareness of human limitations induces us to search for transcendent meaning.

According to the Bible, nature itself holds in its essence a message from the divine to human beings: "Lift up your eyes and see: Who has created these?" (Isa. 40:26). "The heavens proclaim the glory of God, and the firmament announces the work of His hands" (Ps. 19:2). The pandemic is only the latest enigma to challenge and remind us that our search for meaning is ongoing.

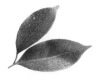

CHAPTER 13

COVID-19 and the Three Dialogues

Each of us, to be fully human, must develop the ability to relate to everyone and everything around us. We are made for this.

From the moment we are born, the dialogue of words and gestures with our parents and family, with whom we interact from our earliest childhood, teaches us interpersonal skills that will be important factors in shaping our personality and adulthood. As we grow, this dialogue hopefully deepens and expands in us.

The philosopher Martin Buber taught that there are three interrelated types of dialogue that should fill our lives: dialogue with our neighbors, dialogue with nature, and dialogue with God.

Consider the dialogue with others. According to the Masoretic text used in Jewish bibles, the biblical verse that describes how Cain killed his brother Abel is incomplete. It says: "And Cain said to his brother Abel; and when they were in the field, Cain set upon his brother Abel and killed him" (Gen. 4:8). Many Christian bibles have words spoken by Cain to his brother, but the Jewish text does not.[37]

The text does not reveal if Cain said anything at all to his brother. Although the rabbinic commentators raised many different possibilities about what words Cain might have spoken, the silence of the text at least shows that no sincere and constructive dialogue existed between them. It could be said, then, that the absence of dialogue led to the first crime in human history: fratricide.

Without dialogue, it is impossible to know another person. The verb *lada'at*, "to know," is often used in biblical Hebrew to refer to the most intimate expression of love between a man and a woman.[38] It is also used in the text of the prophet Hosea to describe the love between God and the people of Israel: "I will espouse you forever: I will espouse you with righteousness and justice, and with loving-kindness and mercy, and I will espouse you with faithfulness; then you shall know the Lord" (Hos. 2:21-22). But knowledge of the other is acquired only through deep, real dialogue. From such knowledge may then come affection.

Dialogue does not refer to superficial relationships. Rather, it demands getting to know others and cultivating an empathic attitude toward them. It requires us to momentarily set aside our own viewpoint and see life from the other's perspective. To achieve this, we need to develop the ability to dialogue with ourselves as well. We must learn to be self-critical, to acknowledge mistakes we have made, and to resolve to reform everything that limits our ability to love and give ourselves to another.

According to Genesis 32 and 33, on the night before Jacob meets with his brother Esau, after years of separation and animosity and with both brothers prepared to fight, Jacob wrestled with an angel until dawn. As dawn broke, the angel told Jacob to release him, but Jacob demanded a blessing first. The angel replied: your name will no longer be Ya'akov but

Yisra'el because you have contended with divine and human beings and have prevailed. Perhaps this name change from Jacob to Israel reflects a change in the patriarch's personality. The change is seen a few verses later when he and his twin brother hug and kiss one another, and then we discover how the change in Jacob has also affected a change in Esau. When we change ourselves, we might also change our neighbor.

We have all been enduring a great calamity. To contend with this plague, the biblical command to love our neighbors as we love ourselves has taken on supreme, contemporary importance.

The pandemic demanded that we respond with social solidarity. I don't mean only the monetary or physical aid that was extended to those in need, but an attitude of constant commitment to the other. The pandemic required— and requires still—that we take care of ourselves in order not to infect others and to care for the other in order to heal our communities. This principle has demonstrably reduced the contagion everywhere that it has been observed. If this practice were to extend to all aspects of life, we would approach the ideals of solidarity that the Bible teaches us through its commandments and regulations, summarized best in Leviticus 19:18: "You shall love your neighbor as yourself."

Then there is the dialogue with nature. Nature constantly communicates messages to us that we must learn to perceive. The Bible regularly refers to this, as in the declaration in Psalm 8:2, "O Lord, our Lord, how majestic is Your name through-out the earth!" Our dialogue with nature leads us to discover its complex and orderly structure, suggesting the presence of a Great Builder who shaped it. It also suggests the need for us to respect and care for the great habitation in which we dwell, both for ourselves and for the generations to come.

The earth cares for us by giving us its fruits for our food. When God created human beings in the biblical narrative, their mission was to tend and till the Garden of Eden (Gen. 2:15). In the same way, we care for the earth by allowing it every seven years to rest from agricultural cultivation for a year (Lev. 25:1-7). Likewise, we find the proscription not to destroy fruit trees in times of war (Deut. 20:19). These rules reflect an aspect of our dialogue with nature.

Finally, the Bible describes the dialogue of human beings with their Creator. The Creator's image is primarily evidenced in each person's actions, and in the relationships we maintain with those around us. In order to dialogue with God, it is essential to have acquired the ability to dialogue with other people.

Leviticus 19:18 literally says: "You shall not avenge yourself or bear a grudge against the sons of your people, but you will love your neighbor as yourself. I am the Lord." The verse links love of neighbor with love for God. This was the understanding of the great Rabbi Akiva, which is why he considered the norm of love for one's neighbor to be an adequate summary of all the commandments in the Torah.[39] In a slightly different way, in the New Testament Gospels, Jesus put love of God ahead of human love when he cited two biblical verses—the one that commands love of God (Deut. 6:5) and the one that commands love of neighbor (Lev. 19:18)—as a summary of all the provisions of the Torah.[40] There is a slight difference between these approaches, but their similarities show us the shared fundamental principles of Christianity and Rabbinic Judaism.

The fact that Jews and Christians hold many essential ideas in common is also seen in Pope Francis's recent encyclical, *Fratelli Tutti*. Pope Francis writes there:

The recent pandemic enabled us to recognize and appreciate once more all those around us who, in the midst of fear, responded by putting their lives on the line. We began to realize that our lives are interwoven with and sustained by ordinary people valiantly shaping the decisive events of our shared history: doctors, nurses, pharmacists, storekeepers and supermarket workers, cleaning personnel, caretakers, transport workers, men and women working to provide essential services and public safety, volunteers, priests and religious....They understood that no one is saved alone.[41]

This is beautifully expressed.

In particular, Pope Francis's *Fratelli Tutti* shows that Jews and Christians share the legacy of the Hebrew prophets. We differ in certain perceptions of God, but we are both committed to a vision of unity, freedom, and love for all human beings, regardless of their particularities and distinctions. He says:

We need to develop the awareness that nowadays we are either all saved together, or no one is saved. Poverty, decadence and suffering in one part of the earth are a silent breeding ground for problems that will end up affecting the entire planet.[42]

A commitment to this vision is what we must cling to in difficult times. Indeed, it is the only way to surmount a crisis.

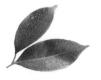

CHAPTER 14

Just Another Crisis?

It seems that after each great catastrophe takes place in human history, we wake up to a new reality and realize that we need to be sure not to repeat the conditions that led to the disaster.

This happened after the Second World War. On October 24, 1945, the United Nations was founded. On December 10, 1948, the United Nations General Assembly, in its Resolution 217 A (III), adopted in Paris the Universal Declaration of Human Rights. These were the first steps to avoid a repetition of the horrors of World War II.

At about the same time, Jewish and Catholic intellectuals, including Jules Isaac and Jacques Maritain, perceived that the centuries-old adversarial relationship between Jews and Christians had contributed to the rise of anti-Semitism and laid the foundations for one of the most horrific crimes in human history: the Shoah. In 1947, they worked with others to convene the Emergency Conference on Anti-Semitism, held in the Swiss town of Seelisberg. The statement released by the delegates of this conference eventually helped to bring about the promulgation in 1965 of the Second Vatican Council document *Nostra Aetate*, the most important step ever toward improved understanding between Jews and Catholics.

There were plenty of other crises. For example, the world divided again in the Cold War between the United States and the Soviet Union. This went on to be a disaster of many decades, without any clear remedies. It, in turn, gave way in the 1990s to a different world after the collapse of the Soviet Union. Several nations were formed in its wake with bright optimism, but then, in many places, this led to the rise of nationalism and more open conflicts.

The September 11, 2001, terrorist attacks on the United States became another watershed moment of terror and heartache, ushering in another new reality. Getting on an airplane, traveling internationally, and entering or leaving the United States, in particular, would never again be the same. A generalized feeling of anxiety took hold in people's hearts, and conflict between established governments and terror groups multiplied exponentially. I wonder if those undeclared wars will ever cease.

Seen in the light of these events, all within my lifetime, the recent pandemic may appear to simply be the latest great upheaval in global stability. Certainly, it spread precipitously and universally, matching the worst projections made for it. We had first waves, second waves, and third waves. Most nations had more than one period of strict quarantine regimens. We've had variants, and these will continue. We also have vaccines, and next, we will have booster shots for those vaccines. There are unforeseen complications and lingering afflictions that beset some of those who have recovered from the disease's worst symptoms.

It seems that history has thrown down the gauntlet to humanity once again. Jewish tradition compels us to ask: Will we learn from the past?

Most of us are unable to offer swift or sweeping solutions to global problems and catastrophes in the way that world leaders might do. But we can all support the spirit and possibility of change. Every crisis deserves and demands a powerful recovery.

The biblical-Talmudic tradition teaches that we all possess the ability to change. Transgressors can always abandon their transgressions and transform themselves into new beings, changing for the better of all. The main cry of the prophets to those who work iniquity is to give up their attitudes and wrong-doings, since it is in the capacities of every human being to transform into a better person. Before dying, Moses, in his last lesson to his people, taught them that life and death, blessing and curse, are forever before them, and they will have to choose life (Deut. 30:19). This is the constant choice possible for each of us.

The process of contrition *(t'shuvah)* that every Jew must carry out, especially in the days before and after the beginning of each year, must lead them to transform into a new being, a better one, through a process of introspection. For instance, at the end of the N'ilah, the closing prayer of the Yom Kippur liturgy, many of us say:

> O Lord our God, out of love You have given us this Yom Kippur to end it in forgiveness of all our sins in order that we cease all acts of exploitation or oppression and turn to You to fulfill your gracious laws with our whole heart.

Change can happen, and positive change is what ought to occur as we emerge from yet another global peril. Will we intentionally seek, in a spirit of solidarity, the health and prosperity of others and not merely struggle for the survival of our own families or nations? Will we forgive those who need forgiveness and work together in order not to repeat the sins of the past?

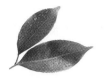

CHAPTER 15

Solidarity with the Weak

The biblical city of Sodom is one of the symbols of evil in the scriptures.[43] From Genesis 19, it can be inferred that the evil of the citizens of Sodom was especially rooted in their desire to dominate others, especially palpable in their practice of sexually brutalizing the vulnerable and weak.

There is a noteworthy mention of Sodom when Ezekiel, speaking prophetically in the voice of God, chastises the city of Jerusalem in his time:

> This was the guilt of your sister Sodom: she and her daughters had pride, excess of food, and prosperous ease, but they did not aid the poor and needy. They were haughty and did abominable things before me; therefore, I removed them when I saw it. (Ezek. 16:49-50)

Ezekiel characterizes the behavior of the inhabitants of Sodom (and other cities, including Jerusalem) as atrocious because the arrogance fostered by their opulent lifestyles made them contemptuous of the destitute.

There has been much discussion over the centuries among Jewish writers about the nature of Sodom's evil. The sages of the Talmud understood that the disgrace of Sodom was manifold, having both bodily and larcenous aspects.[44] The Aramaic translation of the Bible, called Targum Yerushalmi (or Targum Pseudo-Jonathan) explained that Sodom's crime was primarily sexual (Gen. 19:5), as did Rashi (Rabbi Shlomo Yitzchaki), among the classical exegetes of the Middle Ages.

Rashi, Rashbam, (Raabi Shmuel ben Meir) and Ibn Ezra (Rabbi Abraham ben Meir Ibn Ezra), in commenting on the same verse, explained that the neighbors' demand that Lot hand over the strangers he was harboring was to sexually denigrate them.

> The men of the city, the men of Sodom, both young and old, all the people to the last man, surrounded the house; and they called to Lot, "Where are the men who came to you tonight? Bring them out to us, so that we may know them." (Gen. 19:4-5)

Rabbi David Kimhi, for his part, understood their motive to be murderous, while Nachmanides, following the Talmudic approach, interprets that the sin of the inhabitants of Sodom was to murder all those who came to the city because they did not want to share their wealth with anyone else.

All of these explanations go beyond a literal reading of the Genesis narrative, however, especially in relation to their administration of justice. It should be kept in mind that the threat against Lot's visitors is only one example of the crimes of the Sodomites. As Genesis 18:20 recounts: "Then the Lord said: 'How great is the outcry against Sodom and Gomorrah and how very grave their sin!'"

Therefore, it is important to emphasize the nature of the accusations that Ezekiel makes against the conduct of the inhabitants of Sodom: their callousness toward the poor and needy. Considering social injustice as sinful implicates not only the very fabric of human societies but also the individuals within them. Disregard for the needy leads to their isolation from the community and the stratification of society into hierarchical classes. The vulnerable are then treated by the elites as exploitable and disposable.

Moments of crises, such as the COVID-19 pandemic, lay bare the sins of societies that do not care about its weakest members.

All discrimination, whatever its reason—economic, ethnic, or religious—leads to the objectification of the other. It was the fantasy of racial superiority that legitimated the buying and selling of Africans in the New World from the fourteenth to the nineteenth centuries. The devaluation of the human dignity of minority groups, created by the hegemony of those in power, led to the great massacres of the twentieth century, culminating in the Shoah, in which six million people were industrially eliminated for the mere fact of being Jews. The death toll from the centuries of the slave trade will never be known for certain, but there are some estimates as high as sixty million souls. And we know that a slave trade and the dislocation of human populations continue today.

There have been scenes worthy of Sodom during the months of this pandemic. On the other hand, there were many acts of solidarity and great concern for others. There were those who took advantage of the crisis to promote their own miserable interests, but also those who, like Lot in Sodom, opened the doors of their homes to those in need.

When Lot saw them, he rose to meet them, and bowed down with his face to the ground. He said, "Please, my lords, turn aside to your servant's house and spend the night, and wash your feet; then you can rise early and go on your way." (Gen. 19:1-2)

These are the images of a constant struggle between solidarity and selfishness, good and evil. Our responsibility as Jews, or simply as human beings, is to create a society in which there are no longer weak and vulnerable people.

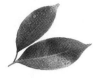

CHAPTER 16

The Loneliness

One of the devasting effects of the pandemic was the frequent necessity of dying alone. Following regulations necessary to hinder the proliferation of the virus, thousands and thousands of people were forced to live in sickness and then die without the comfort of family or friends. It is heartbreaking not to be present with loved ones for a last goodbye or to accompany their remains to the site of their eternal rest.

This plague has caused countless people to endure many moments of loneliness, many of them much more ordinary than death. The silence, melancholy, and uncertainty have also been overwhelming. Ordinarily, we race around from task to task, from activity to activity. During the pandemic, suddenly, we had too much time. We were constrained to look at ourselves in the mirror: confronting our pasts, grappling with frustrations, and examining our masks and facades.

The Bible tells us about two special moments of solitude and reflection in the life of the third patriarch, Jacob. The first was when he left his parents' house for the birthplace of his grandfather Abraham. Jacob fled from the conflict with his brother Esau, a conflict to which his parents had contributed. Then, he was alone. Upon reaching "a certain place," as Genesis

28:11 puts it, he decided to spend the night there. According to rabbinic tradition, it was the same place where Abraham had been ordered to sacrifice his son Isaac (Gen. 22); where Isaac had prayed as the caravan approached with Rebecca, his wife-to-be (Gen. 24:62); and where the Temple of Jerusalem would later be built.[45]

On this occasion, Jacob dreamed of a ladder that united the heavens with the earth. In his utter loneliness, he came to understand the spiritual challenge that was placed before him by his father's blessing to him upon his departure:

> May God Almighty bless you and make you fruitful and numerous that you may become a community of peoples. May He give to you the blessing of Abraham, to you and your offspring with you, so that you may take possession of the land where you now live as an alien—that God gave to Abraham. (Gen. 28:3-4)

The second moment in which Jacob found himself alone was years later. It was the night before he finally encountered his brother again after their long estrangement. Fear and doubt overcame him. Would his brother, Esau, attack him with the four hundred men he commanded? Would he lose the family that he had garnered in the land of Aram with great difficulty and contention (Gen. 32:1-23)? Jacob sent his wives and maids and eleven children ahead of him across the river Jabbok. And so was left by himself (Gen. 32:24-25).

Suddenly, Jacob found himself fighting with a mysterious being, perhaps an angel in human form, whom he was finally able to defeat as dawn approached. The sages of the Midrash speculated that it was the angel of his brother Esau.[46] Perhaps in his loneliness, Jacob was able to relive the conflicts of his past and find healing. Perhaps that nighttime experience enabled him to be hugged and kissed by his brother when they met later that day (Gen. 33:4).

On the one hand, loneliness can lead us to look inward, demanding that we reconsider our lives, what we have received from our ancestors, and what the future ought to be. On the other hand, loneliness can be an inescapable nightmare if the past contains pains that we are unable to face.

Loneliness allowed Moses (Exod. 3), Elijah (1 Kgs. 19:1-18), and probably all the prophets to enter into dialogue with God. In their solitude, they heard the voice of God, more with their hearts and minds than with their ears. God was revealed to Elijah through a soft voice of silence (1 Kgs. 19:12). The psalmist felt and understood the importance of silence in praising God (Ps. 65:2, according to Rashi's interpretation *ad locum*).

People today seem to want to escape from silence for fear of loneliness. When we are alone, we may listen to music or leave the television on in order to feel less alone. Do we want to get away from the small voice of our conscience? Perhaps this has always been the case. Perhaps only a few people are able to endure silence and solitude. The famous Argentine writer Ernesto Sábato was a man who searched for the meaning of existence. Holding a doctorate in physics from the University of La Plata, he abandoned the study of the constitution of the universe in order to probe the human soul. In his first book, *Uno y el Universo (One and the Universe)*, he wrote: "One embarks for distant lands, or pursues human knowledge, or inquires into nature, or seeks God; later it is noticed that the ghost being chased was oneself."[47]

Loneliness and silence lead many to confront the "ghost" of themselves, but it is a reality that can be both heartbreakingly disturbing and energizingly transformative. We should try not to be afraid.

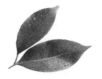

CHAPTER 17

In the Shadow of the Golem

In the April 25, 1953, issue of *Nature*, James Watson and Francis Crick reported on the double-helix structure of DNA for the first time. It was a particularly important step in understanding the molecule that encodes the information that guides the development and biological functioning of all living beings.

Scientific knowledge about DNA has greatly expanded since that early description of its shape. The identification of genes led to the ability to edit them, and so genetic engineering was born. Some of the vaccines against COVID-19 that have been developed have used RNA (DNA's molecular cousin).

The new ability of humans to manipulate genes has given rise to many ethical questions. In 2001, I published an article in the Buenos Aires newspaper *La Nación* outlining my perspectives—based on Jewish sources—on this conflicted and delicate issue. Entitled "In the Shadow of the golem," it came back to my mind as the pandemic wreaked its death and despair, and as a solution to the scourge was desperately sought. The lesson of the golem is still pertinent today.

The idea that it is possible to create living beings out of particular materials through the use of magic formulas has been around since ancient times in many cultures. The Talmud tells us:

> Rava once created a man, a golem, using forces of sanctity. Rava sent his creation before Rabbi Ze'ira [3rd century]. Rabbi Ze'ira wanted to speak to him, but he would not reply. Rabbi Ze'ira said to him: You were created by one of the members of the group, one of the Sages. Return to your dust.[48]

In the early modern age, Philippus Aureolus Theophrastus Bombastus von Hohenheim (1493-1541), who is better known by his pseudonym Paracelsus, was a physician, alchemist, philosopher, and the father of toxicology. He wrote:

> Let the semen of a man putrefy by itself in a sealed cucurbite with the highest putrefaction of the *venter equinus* [horse manure] for forty days, or until it begins at last to live, move, and be agitated, which can easily be seen. After this time, it will be in some degree like a human being, but, nevertheless, transparent and without body. If now, 22 after this, it be every day nourished and fed cautiously and prudently with the arcanum of human blood, and kept for forty weeks in the perpetual and equal heat of a *venter equinus*, it becomes, thenceforth a true and living infant, having all the members of a child that is born from a woman, but much smaller. This we call a homunculus; and it should be afterwards educated with the greatest care and zeal, until it grows up and begins to display intelligence.[49]

This is the famous homunculus or "little man" theory!

A contemporary of Paracelsus was Rabbi Judah Loew ben Bezalel of Prague (c. 1525-1609), known in rabbinical literature by his acronym, Maharal. Vast was his knowledge in rabbinical sources as well as in mathematics, philosophy, and astronomy. He was also a close friend of the astronomer Tycho Brahe. However, the fame of the Maharal is mostly due to his interest in creating a clay golem.

The Hebrew word *golem* means "formless matter" or "raw material." It is found only once in the Hebrew Bible, in Psalm 139:16: "Your eyes saw my unformed body; all the organs of my body were written in Your book; in due time they were formed, to the very last one of them."[50] According to a second- or third-century rabbinic commentary on this verse, *golem* must be understood as a human being in the process of being fashioned by God.

Legend tells us that in order to defend his fellow Jews from the persecutions they were suffering, the Maharal created that clay golem. He placed in the golem's mouth a paper on which the ineffable name of God was written and engraved the word *emet* ("truth" in Hebrew) on the golem's forehead. One day, the golem escaped from the rabbi's control. The Maharal chased after him and, after many attempts, was able to remove the paper from his mouth and erase the first letter of the *emet* from his forehead, leaving the Hebrew word *met*, which means "dead." The golem then decomposed and became clay again. The legend ends by saying that the golem's remains are in the attic of the Altneuschul synagogue in Prague, well out of sight of mortals.

Most of all, golem legends are about the dangers that could threaten humanity when advances in science and technology are used by the unscrupulous.

Knowledge in and of itself is neither good nor bad. Scientific achievements are the products of the inventive human spirit, a manifestation—according to the biblical understanding—of the divine breath that enlivens human beings (Gen. 2:7). The danger is within human beings. It lies within those who give free rein to their excessive ambitions and transform their world into a place where life does not deserve more respect than that which greed allows.

Investigating the molecular structure of what constitutes life or entering into the process of human gestation to correct malformations or diseases are not seen in Judaism as acts in defiance of God. The Talmud teaches: "If the righteous wanted to, they would be able to create a world."[51] Knowledge in the hands of the just is a creative tool that allows humanity to associate with God in the perennial process of recreating the cosmos. However, when everything is easily objectified and commodified, such knowledge can reduce human beings into mere carriers of genetic codes. There lurks the evil of racism. Now that human intellect allows us to edit the very building blocks of life, we must grow in our understanding of each other's spiritual worth or we risk turning everyone into *g´lamim* (the plural of *golem*).

The shadow of the old Prague golem lies behind us, warning us to take heed.

I finished my article from twenty years ago by emphasizing the doubts that plagued me about the use of genetic engineering knowledge in the future. Would genetic weapons be created to destroy enemies in conflict? Or would genetic engineering only be applied to save those affected by the multiple diseases that afflict human beings? The origin of COVID-19 is not known for certain. No one can assure us that it was not created, or that it was not an unpredictable by-product of a laboratory that passed its security filters. But we do know for sure that several of the vaccines achieved were thanks to scientific knowledge of genetic engineering.

Like the knowledge we obtained when scientists manipulated nuclear energy, it is the implementation of that knowledge that makes all the difference in the world. The words of Moses continue to warn us, not only the Hebrews, but all of humanity: "This day I call the heavens and the earth as witnesses against you that I have set before you life and death, the blessing and the curse. And you will choose life, so that you and your children may live" (Deut. 30:19).

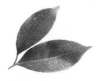

CHAPTER 18

Pandemic and Polemic

One might have hoped that the pandemic would have united all people and their leaders in a common effort to contain and overcome it. Instead, the vituperation on the lips of political leaders seems only to increase.

This makes me think of biblical episodes when a person's offensive words caused them to suffer physically. A rabbinic text comments that the arm of Moses was temporarily afflicted with leprosy (Exod. 4:6-7) because he had slandered the children of Israel by claiming that they would not believe the message that God had commanded him to bring to them (Exod. 4:1).[52]

Later, Moses's sister, Miriam, was struck with leprosy when she and her brother Aaron spoke harshly against Moses's leadership. She had to dwell outside the camp for seven days (Num. 12:1-15). Some rabbis also argued that Aaron experienced the same affliction and for the same reason.[53]

Something similar happens in the story of the leprosy suffered by Na'aman, the chief of the armies of the king of Aram (2 Kgs. 5). When a servant of the prophet Elisha lies about eliciting gifts from the healed Na'aman, he himself is struck with the disease. Thus, the sages of the Talmud interpreted the

Hebrew word that designates the leper, *metzor'a*, as an acronym of *motzi shem r'a*, someone who insults and slanders.[54]

These incidents echo the saying in Proverbs 18:21, "Death and life are in the power of the tongue, and those who love it will eat its fruits."

Words can serve as a devastating weapon, like a deadly arrow. Jeremiah said: "Their tongue is a sharpened arrow, they use their mouths to deceive. One speaks to his fellow in friendship but lays an ambush for him in his heart" (Jer. 9:7).

It is with words of falsehood and infamy that leaders of the past and present have inserted lurid ideas into the minds and hearts of many people. These multiply hatred and demonize the victims they are to hunt down and annihilate. The concentration camps built by Nazism had their origins in the countless speeches of Hitler, in the preaching of Goebbels, and in the filthy pamphlets of Streicher. The beginning of the road leading to Auschwitz was paved with words.

The sages of the Midrash did not see slander as the only offense punishable by leprosy. Those who engaged in paganism, aberrant sexual behavior, the shedding of blood, the desecration of the name of God, cursing God, stealing communal or private property, arrogant behavior, or failed to help others in need were all liable to this penalty.[55]

Perhaps, the sense of this midrashic opinion is that according to the fabric of nature itself, one who does not behave properly will suffer in their body the consequences of their spiritual deterioration. By extension, societies that are led by slanderous rulers end up being devastated.

PART THREE

Emerging into Daylight

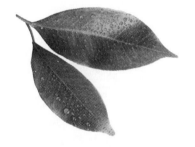

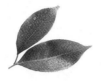

CHAPTER 19

Overcoming Diseases in Dialogue with God

I remember the day in early December 2020 when the United Kingdom began the mass vaccination of its population. The first vaccination day in the US was one week later. Impatiently awaited vaccines seemed to have been achieved in multiple ways by different laboratories using different techniques. Their efficacy was soon confirmed, and people in the UK, US, and elsewhere throughout the world were well on their way to overcoming an insidious disease.

In the ancient world of the Bible, plagues were understood to be sent by God. Even so, there are biblical stories about people who, through their actions, stopped a rampaging disease. For instance, Moses and Aaron intervened when God sent a plague upon participants in the revolt of Korah. By offering incense to God, Aaron made atonement for the people, and the plague subsided (Num. 17:11-14). Similarly, a plague erupted when the Israelites prostituted themselves with the daughters of the Midianites by joining in the worship of their god Ba'al Pe'or. Phinehas, the grandson of Aaron, stopped that epidemic by killing an Israelite man and the Midianite woman he was with (Num. 25:1-15).

Psalm 106 recalls this incident:

They attached themselves to Baʻal Peʻor, ate sacrifices offered to pagan idols.

They provoked anger by their deeds, and a plague broke out among them.

Phinehas stood up and intervened, and the plague ceased.

It was reckoned to his merit from generation to generation, to eternity.

(Ps. 106:28-31)

But the psalmist only speaks of Phinehas interceding with God, apparently through prayer.

Reading these biblical passages from the perspective of the twenty-first century offers another understanding. God's greatest creation, the human species, is gifted with a powerful intellect. People are not passive beings who only act according to instinctive impulses or behave only in a repetitive, automaton-like manner. Humans are thus becoming able to use science to develop genetic tools to combat the deadly viruses caused by random mutations in nature.

But a biblical worldview would insist there is an ongoing dynamic between the Creator and humanity. The intensifying human mastery of the world must be accompanied by the spiritual growth that results from a constant dialogue with the Creator. Like parents and their children, this dialogue involves arguments, challenges, and rapt listening to one another.

According to the Bible, we live in a state of duality. On the one hand, God gave us the power to dominate the earth. On the other hand, God prohibited the intake of the fruit of the tree of knowledge of good and evil. (See Genesis 1:27-28.) The human being has an enormous capacity that manifests through creativity in science and technology. However, there is always a limit to the development of our abilities.

The same duality can be found in two verses of the book of Psalms. On the one hand, it says: "The heavens belong to the Lord, but the Earth was given to man" (Ps. 115:16), and on the other, "The earth belongs to the Lord and everything in it" (Ps. 24:1).

The sages of the Talmud explain that the land and the fruits are of God, but when saying a blessing before making use of them, it is as if we acquired them.[56] In other words, to us was given the ability to act on the Creator's work, provided that we know before Whom we are working.

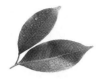

CHAPTER 20

Light in the Darkness

As news of available vaccines began to cheer the hearts of many, the candles of the Hanukkah festival were being lit. Hanukkah commemorates the reopening of the Temple in Jerusalem by the Hasmoneans on the twenty-fifth of Kislev, 165 BCE, when the holy menorah within its complex was relit. This candelabrum was the trophy paraded by the Romans who destroyed that sanctuary in 70 CE, as can be seen to this day in the bas-relief on the Arch of Titus in the Forum in Rome.

The menorah held a place of special sanctity within the Temple, as evidenced by windows that allowed the interior light to shine to the outside but prevented exterior light from entering inside (1 Kgs. 6:4). Rabbinic midrash explains that this physical arrangement symbolized the world's need for the menorah's sacred light, while the holy place had no need of the world's light.[57] Likewise, when the priest lit the menorah, the light from its six arms had to focus on the central candle, indicating that it served to provide light for humanity since God did not need such illumination.[58]

A link between the candle and the individual is presented in two verses of the Book of Proverbs: "For the commandment [of God] is a lamp and the Torah a light" (Prov. 6:23) and

"The human spirit is the lamp of the Lord" (Prov. 20:27). The lamp refers both to the individual Jew and to the Jewish people because that light gave testimony to the fact that the Divine Presence abided in Israel.[59] Moreover, although it was normally the priests who prepared and lit the menorah in the Temple, any Jew could also light it.[60]

Inspired by the two verses quoted above from the book of Proverbs, Shimon bar Kappara', one of the sages of the Talmud of the late second and early third centuries, taught:

> Both the human being and the Torah were compared to a candle; it is as if God told to each individual: my candle, the Torah, is in your hands, and your candle, your life, in mine. Take care of mine, and I'll take care of yours.[61]

From this, we can conclude that in the same way that light allows us to see everything around us, we should also look for the light that enlightens our inner spirit, and our brain has the ability to process it. But this cognitive work requires the light that emanates from the values that reflect justice, equity, goodness, and love. So the process of human knowledge leads to the construction of a reality that dignifies the human condition.

When the Romans destroyed the Temple in 70 CE, they may have plundered the menorah, but they could not steal its fire. So it is that today, on every evening during Hanukkah, a new candle is lit, until, after eight days, all the candles are shining. Although many explanations of this practice exist, foremost in my mind is that this fire demands all who see it to keep ever in mind the virtues of hope and faith.

We desperately need and seek a light to illuminate the darkness. May the message of the Hanukkah candles give us encouragement—this year and every year—to light our way.

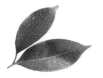

CHAPTER 21

Reflections on Redemption as Christians Celebrate the Nativity

Redemption *(g'ulah)* and salvation *(y'shu'ah)* are among the concepts in the Bible central to the faiths of both Jews and Christians. I know there are many Jews and Christians, both, who have been pondering these concepts in light of the life-threatening pandemic. It is no small wonder to contemplate what it means to be saved or redeemed when we also feel that our everyday lives are at risk.

The terms *g'ulah* and *y'shu'ah* are often casually used interchangeably, but there are certain distinctions in the Jewish tradition worth noting. While salvation refers to the liberation of a human being from the oppression inflicted on them by another (Exod. 14:13; Ps. 14:7), or oppression inherent in the drama of the human condition (Ps. 62:2), redemption seems to allude to a return to an ideal past situation that was impaired or lost.

In Leviticus 25, the word *g'ulah* is applied to the return or redemption of property to its original owners. This would re-establish the Hebrew vision of an ideal society in which land or property was equitably divided among families to make them self-sufficient. Also, in Jewish understanding, redemption, although it ultimately comes from God, requires the collaborative efforts of God and humanity. God revealed to Moses the divine intention to redeem the children of Israel from Egypt and restore their freedom (Exod. 6:6), but this plan would require Moses to encourage the Hebrew people to leave the land of their enslavement.

In contrast, salvation is a revelation or deed of the Creator in which Jews must place their faith and hope. The Talmud describes six questions that the heavenly tribunal asks each Jew who has died.[62] One of them is: "Did you believe and wait for God's salvation?" Note that salvation must be awaited while redemption must be actively pursued.

The concept of an anointed Messiah to advance God's plans is also relevant here. In some Jewish interpretations, Isaiah 11 is the first time in which the idea of a future Messiah appears in the Bible in reference to a king of Israel. This individual is envisioned as a descendant of David who will reign in a time of justice and universal knowledge of God. In the following chapter, Isaiah speaks about salvation. In these passages, we can see the intimate relationship between the two words *Mashi'ach* and *y'shu'ah* (Messiah and salvation).

Over time, messianic thinking became linked to the inter-pretation of both salvation and redemption. It was discussed within Judaism both before and after the time of Jesus. Some passages in the Dead Sea Scrolls refer to multiple messiahs,[63] and a unique fragment seems to refer to a Messiah raising the dead.[64] The Talmud presents yet different opinions about the coming of this figure.[65]

When Christians prepare to celebrate the birth of Jesus of Nazareth, it might be good to recall that his name undoubtedly derives from *Y'shu'a*, meaning "God saves" or "God save!" and that it has messianic connotations. Indeed, over the centuries, the question of whether the Messiah had already come or was still awaited divided Jews and Christians into antagonistic camps. Barriers of misunderstanding were erected. Political, economic, and social factors promoted a relationship of animosity between them, with the result that there was little incentive to seek the path of dialogue.

As Pope Francis has said, a new "journey of friendship" between both communities has begun in our time, thanks to *Nostra Aetate* and the continuing efforts of all those who labor to transform that document into a living reality. I know that this is an ongoing effort in the Roman Catholic Church worldwide, and that many Christians, Catholic or not, are turning away from earlier beliefs that Jewish people need saving; in other words, that we require a Christian understanding of salvation. Since *Nostra Aetate*, Catholics and other Christians are, instead, beginning to see that the redemption and salvation of the Jews were presupposed in the teachings of Jesus and the early church.

We can now learn from each other that, in our different ways, Jews and Christians both await the fullness of salvation for all of Creation.

From the Jewish perspective, the concept of redemption demands and compels us both to work together to correct, with the help of the Eternal, that which has gone astray. The pandemic, economic crises, widespread racism and divisiveness, and rampant hunger and homelessness all demand that we seek to redeem the situation and labor to restore the world to God's intentions for it. In this understanding of the process of redemption, human beings have an active role, because according to the Sages, by acting with justice and righteousness, they become God's partner in completing the creation of the cosmos.[66]

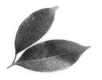

CHAPTER 22

Being at Home

At many points during the successive waves of this pandemic, various countries declared national lockdowns in an effort to contain the virus and keep their citizens safe. People found themselves having to stay inside their homes for long periods, a situation that psychologically upset many. There were increases in family violence as well as depression, which not only increased but sometimes went untreated. This distress occurred in many countries and was not restricted to specific cultures.

As we emerge into the daylight, it would be good to reestablish the meaning of being at home.

Home used to be the refuge that sheltered people from all the turmoil and conflicts of the outside world. It was the family domain where, despite any internal tensions, a common bond would hopefully unite its members in safety and security. I was blessed to grow up in this type of home during my childhood in Buenos Aires. I lived in an immigrant community. The parents or grandparents who had fled from turmoil, war, and persecution in Europe or the Middle East came to Argentina in the hopes of building a better future for themselves and their children. It was a brave and daring journey to leave loved ones behind in order to build new lives in a strange land with a strange language and a strange culture.

One of the characteristics of our times is a trend to turn the home into a luxury residence. What were once refuges and havens often seem transformed into hotels occupied by individuals who share less time together and have weaker ties of affection. Ample individual spaces, personal entertainment devices, and a seeming lack of need for human connection often dominate. This is not at all like what home meant when I was a child or even when I was raising my children.

The pandemic caused a reassessment of the importance of the home as both a shelter and a workplace, for those who can do their jobs remotely. In other words, our idea of home has been rapidly changing!

In Jewish tradition, home is the primary place for the transmission of Jewish culture and identity. The reason why traditional Judaism only accepts marriages between Jews as religiously legal is precisely because of the educational and formative importance of life within the family. Some rabbinic texts suggest that Jewish identity is passed on to children by their mother because of her traditional role as the primary shaper of her children's character:

> The Gemara asks: From where do we deduce that betrothal with a gentile woman is legally ineffective? From the verse: "Neither shall you make marriages with them" [Deut. 7:3], which teaches that marrying gentile women is meaningless halachically [according to Jewish law]. The Gemara asks: We have found that betrothal is legally ineffective with her; from where do we derive that her offspring is like her?

Rabbi Yochanan says in the name of Rabbi Shimon bar Yochai: As the verse states with regard to the same issue: "Your daughter you shall not give to his son… for he will turn away your son from following Me" [Deut. 7:3-4]. Since the verse refers to the case of a Jewish daughter that marries a gentile, it is the gentile who will lead his child away from the service of God; this indicates that "your son" in the verse refers to your grandson. Hence the offspring from a Jewish woman is called "your son" by the Torah, but your son from a gentile woman is not called your son, but her son.[67]

Since in ancient times, the man was the economic breadwinner of the family, the woman was in charge of the home. For this reason, we find the following reflection in the Talmud:

Rabbi Yosei said: "In all my days, I did not call my wife, my wife; nor my ox, my ox. Rather, I called my wife, my home [because she is the pillar] of the home; and my ox, my field (because it is the primary force in the fields).[68]

In Genesis 1:28, God tells human beings to "be fruitful and multiply." When the sages of the Talmud wondered how many children a man must have in order to fulfill God's command, the house of Hillel said: "A male and a female, as it is stated: 'Male and female God created them' [Gen. 5:2]."[69] From this it follows that just as human beings must imitate God in their lives, in the same way that God created the cosmos and put in it a complete Adam, that is, a man and a woman, the same must be done by each family through the creation of a microcosm that is the home.[70] In the Talmud we read:

The Sages taught: One who loves his wife as he loves himself, and who honors her more than himself, and who leads his sons and daughters in an upright way, and who marries them off near the time when they reach maturity, about him the verse states: And you shall know that your tent is in peace. (Job 5:24)[71]

In the twenty-first century, society sees man, woman, and family in quite different ways from this Talmudic vision. So, too, does much of the Jewish world, as we continue to evolve and interpret meaning in our own time.

But the pandemic has offered us an opportunity to reexamine what is happening in our families and in our homes. Perhaps we will find fresh ways to create nurturing spaces that resemble what home once meant. Perhaps the unwelcome lockdowns we have experienced will encourage us to be more conscientious about cultivating homes that are sanctuaries and safe harbors from the world's tumults. Maybe, as so many of us continue to work from home, we will find good ways to create helpful boundaries between work responsibilities and family activities. There's no question that the spaces in which we live function differently from how they did even just a few years ago

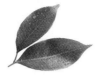

CHAPTER 23

Job-Like Anguish

One of the consequences of the pandemic has been the feeling of anguish experienced by many people worldwide, especially as government leaders took advantage of the crisis to advance their own interests, heedless of collapsing economies and deteriorating social conditions. The loss of income and professions, and comfortable or necessary routines, shortages of essentials, unprecedented restrictions, and deep-seated uncertainties about the future have led many to a state of mind that is well described by the word *anguish*.

The word comes down from Middle English via Old French and is derived from the Latin *angustia*, (narrowness), from *angustus* (narrow). It is interesting to note that the Hebrew word for the same sensation is *tzarah*, from *tzar*,[72] which also means "narrow." One memorable instance of this in the Torah comes in the story of Balaam and his talking donkey: "Once more the angel of the Lord went forward and stood himself on a spot so **narrow** that there was no room to turn right or left" (Num. 22:26). Feeling crushed or stuck in an apparent dead end is an extremely hard experience to bear.

Another memorable appearance of the word, quite different from the first, comes in the Prophets, from Isaiah: "From the west, they shall revere the name of the Lord, and from the east, His Glory. For He shall come like a narrow river which the wind of the Lord drives on" (Isa. 59:19). The intensity of God's power and Presence are compared to the same sort of narrowness.

We find in the Bible different responses to anguish. In Psalms 118:5, we read: "I called upon the Lord in my distress [or 'from a tight place']; The Lord answered me and put me in a wide-open space." Similarly, Psalm 20:2: "May the Lord answer you when you are distressed *[tzarah]*; may the name of the God of Jacob protect you [or 'lift you up']."

The psalmist's response is full faith and hope in God. It is the response of people of faith who do not despair, who constantly struggle in their faith and hope that the Lord will bless their efforts.

A different attitude was adopted by Job, who suddenly lost all his children and his goods. He was totally dispossessed. He sat down to mourn for his deceased children and said: "Naked I came out of my mother's womb and naked I will return there; the Lord has given, and the Lord has taken away; blessed be the name of the Lord" (Job 1:21). When his health fails, his wife tells him to curse God and die (Job 2:9). Job reproaches her for this attitude and continues to maintain his faith in God, despite everything that has happened to him. He does not renounce his active attitude in life; he does not abandon himself or surrender. He does not claim God's help but needs an explanation for his misfortune. He was a just man respectful of the Creator, yet he feels that he was abandoned by Him. He is accompanied by his faithful friends who urge him to meditate on his mistakes since the Lord is always just. Job replies that he does not find in his actions a transgression so serious as to merit such a great punishment.

God finally reveals himself to Job (chapter 38 and following). God's answer is that there is no answer whatsoever that He can provide since the gulf between God and humankind is immeasurable. God also tells Job to offer sacrifices of atonement for his faithful friends, since they pretended to know the intimacy of divine thought (Job 42:7-9). But the account does not appear to offer an answer. Job rebuilds his life with his pain.

Martin Buber finds in the story a subtle answer: "No explanation has been given to us, questions and inquests were not answered, wrong did not become just, malice did not turn into pity. Nothing happened, but the man returned to hear the voice of God calling him again."[73] And that was enough for Job. The last thing necessary for every human being.

Job-like anguish has been experienced by many Jews—and many people, everywhere, of all backgrounds—over the centuries.

For example, the destruction of the Second Temple in Jerusalem in 70 CE was a religious and national catastrophe for the Jewish people. Thousands died in the war against the Romans, and many others were enslaved. A deep sense of anguish seized many. Some responded to this tragedy with a desire to adopt a life of asceticism and avoid any pleasure. Rabbi Yehoshu'a disagreed, arguing that the loss of the Temple must be mourned but that impossible demands should not be placed upon the people. Life must go on.[74]

Anxiety paralyzes. It keeps the afflicted in a state of inaction and vulnerability. The antidote to overcoming this situation is to recreate hope. According to the Midrash, the Messiah was born the same day the Temple was destroyed.[75] Perhaps this can be interpreted to mean that the identity of the Jewish people was not lost because they knew how to recreate their hope from generation to generation, despite the persecutions and massacres they suffered over the following centuries.

In the post-pandemic world, there will be millions of people with feelings of oppression, loss, and anguish. Hope does not mean a delusional or passive attitude. Rather, it means that a person is committed to achieving a goal. Despite the difficulties and losses and scarcities that this pandemic has caused for so many around the world, the recovery of a life of dignity must be the hope clung to by the anguished. Such hope can be the very foundation of our lives.

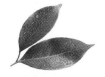

CHAPTER 24

The Pandemic and War

On April 15, 2021, a particularly important meeting organized by the Permanent Mission of the Holy See to the United Nations took place in Geneva. It gathered representatives of international and religious institutions, together with high-ranking Vatican dignitaries, to study the implications of the latest encyclical by Pope Francis, *Fratelli Tutti*. The participants considered it to be an exceptional document, a desperate appeal to all humankind in difficult times, including a devastating pandemic.

When reading the encyclical for the first time, I found myself hoping that its spirit and vision would become a reality; that it would sensitize powerful leaders, whose decisions affect the destinies of billions of people scattered around the globe, to the real needs of human beings and of the planet.

The central focus of *Fratelli Tutti* is the need to care for the world and to inspire its inhabitants to love one another. This is, of course, a defining vision found in many verses of the Hebrew Bible shared by Jews and Christians. The encyclical considers these overarching needs in the context of the global crisis as well as the violent outbursts that set people against one another in various places.

These days—as I write these words now—we are witnessing a new conflict in the Middle East, in which bombs and missiles silence words of peace and reconciliation. The notion of loving one another seems far away, yet again. Who will give life to those who are slain? Who will give back the joy of living to families who lose their loved ones?

The present reality recalls the situation described in the biblical account of the Tower of Babel. Technological progress in building construction allowed the inhabitants of that city to create ever greater structures. Their abilities magnified their arrogance to the point that they sought to challenge God. In consequence, God imposed a confusion of languages upon the builders of the tower. Each person found that they could not understand the language of their neighbors (Gen. 11:7).

And as I said in the book *On Heaven and Earth*: "The Midrash states that what really bothered God was that the builders were more concerned about losing a single brick than with losing a man who might fall from such a great height." The problematic priorities of those ancient builders resemble problems that remain with us today. Cardinal Bergoglio responded then: "When one reads Maimonides and Saint Thomas Aquinas, two nearly contemporary philosophers, we see that they always start by putting themselves in the position of their adversary in order to understand them; they dialogue from the standpoint of the other."[76]

Today the lethal force of weapons technology silences words that can seek to solve conflicts and bring understanding. When missiles and bombs become the language of communication, the only result is more hatred, more division, more death.

Peace must be taught in all the schools of the world as the supreme value to be achieved. It must be the central principle of education everywhere. The sages of the Talmud lifted up the gestures that must be adopted in order to promote the ways of peace, for instance, the help to the poor must include the gentiles. They concluded that the Torah was delivered to the people of Israel so that they could teach others about the paths of peace.[77] And the culmination of the famous priestly blessing is peace: "The Lord lift His favor upon you and grant you peace!" (Num. 6:26).

In the days of the Bible, Jerusalem, at times, knew extreme violence. But the vision of Zechariah 8:3-5 offers a divine perspective:

> Jerusalem will be called the Faithful City, and the mountain of the Lord Almighty will be called the Holy Mountain....There shall yet be old men and women in the squares of Jerusalem, each with a cane in his hand because of their great age. And the squares of the city streets will be crowded with boys and girls playing in the squares there.

This prophecy will materialize when its message, and the message of *Fratelli Tutti*, together with all the yearnings for peace and justice, cease to be mere written letters but become words embedded in our hearts.

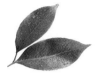

CHAPTER 25

The Pandemic and the Peddler

A complex and difficult period in our shared history is coming to an end. This has been a time unlike any in our memory. It was not like 2001 when the destruction of the World Trade Center in New York made international terrorism a global security priority. Neither have these years been thrown into chaos because of extreme economic cycles. The COVID-19 pandemic has been faceless and mindless. It has infected human beings indiscriminately wherever and whenever it can.

Perversion and madness persist in many leaders and members of the great human family. The horrifying scenes of the hundreds of graves opened to bury the victims of the pandemic, of the mass graves, of pain and anguish, seem not to have moved a humanity in which indifference and selfishness prevail over solidarity and empathy. I wish that this were not so; but this is what I see.

In 1943, Shmu'el Yosef Agnon, the only Hebrew-language writer to have been awarded the Nobel Prize in Literature, wrote a short story he called "The Lady and the Peddler." It was first published in Tel Aviv in a collection of writings called *BeSa'ar*

(In the Storm). The volume was edited by the Hebrew Writers Association and dedicated to Jewish soldiers who had served in the British Army to fight Axis troops during the Second World War.

Agnon's story tells about a Jewish peddler who brings his wares to an isolated house deep inside a dense forest. The woman who lives there treats the peddler with contempt and shows no interest in his merchandise until she notices a large knife, like one used by hunters. She purchases it.

Since a blizzard has struck, the peddler asks the woman if he might stay in her barn until the storm passes. A relationship grows between them. The peddler puts aside his Jewish traditions, eats non-kosher foods, and stops praying. The woman prepares hearty meals for him, although she never tastes them herself. When the peddler asks her why she does not eat, she confesses that she eats human flesh and drinks human blood. The Jew backs away from her, perceiving a scent of hunger emanating from her mouth.

That night, the peddler goes further into the forest because he feels a need to pray. When he returns to his straw bed in the barn, he discovers that there are holes in it. He realizes that the woman has tried to stab him in the dark and then finds the woman's corpse. She had mortally wounded herself in her attempt to kill him. The peddler then builds a coffin for her, but because of the heavy snowfall, he cannot bury it.

Reviewers understand that Agnon, in his story, was describing the relationship of Jews with their neighbors in Nazi Germany.[78]

Every time I read this tale, its ending irritates me. The Jew took his belongings and went on his way, hawking his wares.

Many of Agnon's stories feature characters who develop their lives in vicious circles, trapped in situations that dramatically require urgent changes that they fail to make. Like this peddler, who had more and more clear evidence of the danger that his life was in yet did not immediately leave that house of horror in which he found himself. Having overcome terrible danger, he took his gear and continued on his way. Nothing seems to have affected his life; apparently, he learned nothing from his experience.

I refuse, in this time, to simply return to the status quo, to hawk trinkets, to lose hope.

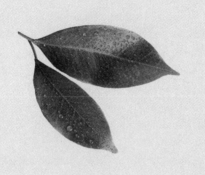

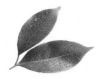

Epilogue

"For though my faith is not yours and your faith is not mine, if we each are free to light our own flame, together we can banish some of the darkness of the world."
— Rabbi Lord Jonathan Sacks

By the time you read this, it will be two years since we became aware of the existence of "the novel coronavirus" and later of its severity. The pandemic caused and still causes suffering. Its complications and consequences will affect us for a long time.

The crisis was not a localized one that the rest of humanity could ignore. Graphic images of people being buried in mass graves or cremated in large groups have flashed across the global electronic media. Our children and grandchildren will have trouble forgetting those images. Many of us suffered the death of a friend or a family member, and many more may still. The separation from loved ones has been unbearable. The damage to the worldwide economy was gigantic.

In a world where resources are squandered, and many people live as if in a disposable society, we suddenly realized that some things—lives, relationships—are invaluable. We have discovered that people we casually encountered and dismissed in everyday life are really essential and valuable. We have experienced, anew, the truth of the old saying, "Money can't buy everything." And we have become painfully aware that we are far from being the masters of our own fates.

Leaders who tried to deny or avoid the crisis caused their people pain, suffering, and the loss of hundreds of thousands of lives. Many businesses and companies, some with long histories, closed their doors forever because they could not endure long and necessary quarantines. Uncertainty pervaded all of life.

It is impossible to contemplate all of the lives, plans, and dreams that this disease has disrupted or ended. We have all been through a terrible storm.

In their daily prayers, Jews recite verse 20 of Psalm 68: "Blessed is the Lord. Day by day God supports us, God, our deliverance." It suggests that while we must plan for the future, we should also thank God for the day that we are currently living.

Rabbi Simcha Bunim Bonhardt of Peshischa taught that life consists of dualities with which we interact throughout our lives. For instance, he said that people should have two pockets in their clothing. In one, there should be a paper on which it is written, "For me, the world was created," and in the second pocket, one reading, "I am dust and ashes" (Gen. 18:27).[79] At certain times we should think of ourselves as the most precious thing in existence, while at other times as an insignificant handful of dust. We must live believing that we are immortal beings and, at the same time, be aware that we are only one step away from death. As David said to Jonathan: "As the Lord lives and as you live, there is but a step between me and death" (1 Sam. 20:3).

Life also teaches us that we must live for the future, striving to realize our aspirations—but at the same time recognize that not everything that happens is under our command. One of the most devastating effects of this pandemic, apart from the all-too-many deaths, has been the terrible loss of control that it carried. Long-planned events had to be postponed or canceled. Dreams were frustrated. Life went on, but a significant part of it was shredded.

Frustration is such a powerful feeling that Isaiah ascribed it even to God when observing the injustices rampant in the prophet's time:

> He dug the ground up, cleared it of stones, and planted it with choice vines. He built a watchtower inside it. He made a wine press therein; for He hoped it would yield grapes. Instead, it yielded wild grapes. (Isa. 5:2)

In the face of frustration, loss of control, uncertainty, and pain, we should aim both to persevere and hope. In the times of the Roman emperor Hadrian, Jews were forbidden to study the Torah. Great spiritual leaders rebelled against the empire. Hadrian's forces captured ten sages, tried them, and then martyred them with horrific torments. Yeshbab the Scribe was one of these. When his students asked what to do, the teacher replied: "Hold on to each other and love peace and justice; maybe there is hope."[80]

Hope is one of the fundamental components of resilience. We see this in numerous biblical passages in the context of the first devastation of Jerusalem in 586 BCE (for example, Isa. 40, Jer. 31:16, Lam. 3:29, Ps. 126). Hope cannot be built upon what has been irreversibly lost. It is (re)built by beginning to create anew. The penultimate verse of Lamentations says: "Restore us to Yourself, Lord, that we may return; renew our days as of old" (Lam. 5:21). The combination of "renewal" and "as of old" contains great teaching. All hope must be both a restoration and a renewal.

After the grief of losing a loved one, it is not possible to return to the reality before the death. Still, one must rebuild life in its fullness, including in it the memory of those who have left us forever.

After the second destruction of Jerusalem in 70 CE, Rabbi Yochanan ben Zakkai summoned the wise men of Israel to restore the Jewish people. His work as a spiritual leader of his time was to maintain continuity with the past and to build a new future—which we see in the gradual development of Rabbinic Judaism. He did not remain paralyzed. He managed to escape being hemmed in besieged Jerusalem and obtained from the Roman general Vespasian space in the city of Yavneh to reconstitute the Sanhedrin (Rabbinical Parliament).[81] The scholars of Yavneh developed new ways to sustain the religious beliefs and practices of the Jewish people in a world without the Temple in Jerusalem. Many of the rituals that could only occur there had to be maintained in temporary new ways until the Sanctuary might be reconstructed.[82] The Temple was not built again, and the transitory became the permanent reality. The life of the Jewish people had continuity with the past but grew into new forms.

The pandemic storm has devasted millions of families and may yet devastate millions more who will have to rebuild their lives, their livelihoods, and their dreams. Pain tends to paralyze us, creating a vicious cycle, since inaction easily plunges us into depression and anguish.

Humanity in our day is called to get up and continue working for a better world. Crises summon us to strengthen ourselves. Poets and musicians create stirring expressions of these imperatives. In the dark days of battling Nazism, for example, the young poet and fighter Hannah Szenes wrote:

My God, My God, I pray that these things never end,
The sand and the sea,
The rustle of the waters,
Lightning of the Heavens,
The prayer of Humanity.[83]

While on a mission to rescue her Jewish brothers and sisters in her homeland of Hungary, Hannah Szenes was betrayed by fascists, then tortured and executed on November 7, 1944. Nonetheless, her song continues to inspire us, along with all those other poems and artworks that touch on the essential aspects of existence.

We are beginning to see the end of the present nightmare. Beyond our pain, frustration, and anguish, and using our God-given gifts for discovery and ingenuity, the gates of a return to a new stability are beginning to open.

Twenty-four centuries ago, the prophet Malachi envisioned a new and ultimate future: "But to you who fear My name, the sun of righteousness will rise with healing in its wings" (Mal. 3:20).

Acknowledgments

Thank you to the publishers and hosts where some of these chapters, in slightly different form, first appeared or were delivered. Chapter 10, "The Days of Awe," was published in the Vatican newspaper, *L'Osservatore Romano*, on September 18, 2020. Chapter 11, "Reflections on an Unusual Yom Kippur," was delivered as a sermon at Temple Beth Hillel-Beth El, Wynnewood, Pennsylvania. Chapter 13, "COVID-19 and The Three Dialogues," is adapted from a talk I gave as an opening address of the Third Congress of Interreligious Dialogue, which I shared with Archbishop Víctor Fernández, and which was held virtually from La Plata, Argentina, on October 21, 2020. An earlier version of Chapter 21, "Reflections on Redemption as Christians Celebrate the Nativity," was published in *L'Osservatore Romano* on December 21, 2020, and chapter 24, "The Pandemic and the War," appeared on May 19, 2021, in *L'Osservatore Romano*.

About the Author

Rabbi Abraham Skorka was born in Buenos Aires, Argentina. He earned a PhD in chemistry from the University of Buenos Aires and graduated from Midrasha HaIvrit and the Latin-American Rabbinical Seminary. He was the rabbi of Benei Tikva Synagogue for forty-two years and rector of the Latin-American Rabbinical Seminary for twenty. He has published many articles and books, including *On Heaven and Earth*, an international bestseller, which he wrote with then-archbishop of Buenos Aires, Cardinal Bergoglio, who is now Pope Francis. Rabbi Skorka has received honorary doctorates from the Pontifical Catholic University of Argentina, the Jewish Theological Seminary, and Sacred Heart University, Fairfield, CN. He has received awards from the legislature of the Autonomous City of Buenos Aires and the Polish Council of Christians and Jews, and the Eternal Light Award from the Center for Catholic-Jewish Studies at Saint Leo University in Florida, as well as the Jan Karski Eagle Award. He recently served a term as a university professor at Saint Joseph's University in Philadelphia, working closely with its Institute for Jewish-Catholic Relations. Currently, he serves as Distinguished Professor of Jewish Studies at Gratz College, Melrose Park, PA. Today, he and his wife make their home in the Philadelphia area, and Rabbi Skorka frequently gives talks on Jewish topics and issues related to Jewish-Catholic relations.

Notes

1   *b. Menachot* 29b.

2   *b. 'Eruvin* 13a.

3   *B'reishit Rabbah* (Albeck-Theodor), *parashat B'reishit, parashah* 20.

4   *b. Shabbat* 33b.

5   *Mishneh Torah, Sefer Hamad'a, Hilchot De'ot* 1-3, *shemonah p'rakim, perek* 4.

6   Joseph Dan, "Gershom Scholem's Reconstruction of Early Kabbalah," *A Journal of Jewish Ideas and Experience* 5, no. 1 (February 1985): 39-66, https://doi.org/10.1093/mj/5.1.39.

7   See, for example, Alvin Toffler, *Future Shock* (1970), and *The Third Wave* (1980).

8   See also Leviticus 26:3-43.

9   See also Jeremiah 12:1-5 and the entire book of Job.

10   1 Samuel 4:17 and 6:4, 2 Samuel 17:9, and Psalms 106:29. See Rashi on Exodus 7:27, D"H (*Dibbur HaMathil* = Referential words): *Hineni Nogef*, and Radak on Genesis 5:24, D"H: *Vaithalekh*.

11   See Numbers 17:6-15 and 25:8, and 2 Samuel 24. See also *m. Avot* 4:15.

12   *m. Avot* 2:16.

13   *b. Menachot* 29b.

14   Erich Fromm, *The Fear of Freedom* (New York: Routledge, 2001) 3. First published in 1942.

15   *m. Avot* 1:14.

16   Herbert A. Davidson, "The Middle Way in Maimonides' Ethics," *American Academy for Jewish Research* 54 (1987): 31-72.

17   *Hilchot Ta'aniyot* 5:12-13, based on *b. Bava Batra* 60b.

18   Ismar Schorsch, "Memory: Judaism's Lifeblood," a reflection for Purim on the JTS website: https://www.jtsa.edu/memory-judaisms-lifeblood.

19   See the classic rabbinic discussion in *b. Sanhedrin* 59b.

20   *b. Sanhedrin* 56a-60a; *t. Avodah Zarah* 8:4. In the *midrashim* they are found in: *B'reishit Rabbah*, chapters 16, 26, 34; *Sh'mot Rabbah*, chapter 30; *B'midbar Rabbah*, chapter 14; *D'varim Rabbah*, chapters 1, 2; *Shir Hashirim Rabbah*, chapter 1; *Kohelet Rabbah*, chapter 2 *Tanchuma, Yitro*, etc. In the Jerusalem Talmud, although the seven Noahide precepts are not mentioned exhaustively, they are referred to on various occasions; for example, *y. Yevamot* 11:2, 12a; *y. Kiddushin* 1:1, 58c.

21 In Talmudic literature, the Jew is referred to on various occasions as *Ben Brit*, "Son of the Covenant," that is, one who is committed to the Covenant; for example: *m. Bava Kamma* 1:2, 3. According to Rashi's reading of Deuteronomy 29:13-14, even future Jewish generations entered into the Covenant with God at Sinai.

22 Yad, *Sefer Shoftim, Hilchot Melachim* 8:11.

23 *The Digest of Justinian, Volume 1*, trans. and ed. Alan Watson (Philadelphia: University of Pennsylvania Press, 1998), 1.1.9, page 2.

24 Vilna edition, 7:13.

25 *b. Avodah Zarah* 53b.

26 *Pirkei DeRabbi Eli'ezer* 24.

27 José Ortega y Gasset, *The Revolt of the Masses*, translated anonymously from the Spanish (New York: W.W. Norton, 1964), 11-12.

28 See Hanoch Ben Pazi, "Messianic Humanism—The Jewish Humanism of André Neher: André Neher in the Footsteps of Martin Buber and Abraham Joshua Heschel," *Daat: A Journal of Jewish Philosophy & Kabbalah*, no. 84 (407-426, (2017 / תשע"ח.

29 *b. Bava Metzi'a* 58b.

30 *Berachot* 8a.

31 Jorge Mario Bergoglio and Abraham Skorka, *On Heaven and Earth: Pope Francis on Faith, Family, and the Church in the Twenty-First Century*, trans. Alejandro Bermudez and Howard Goodman (New York: Image, 2013), 55-56.

32 *m. Berachot* 4:4.

33 *b. Berachot* 7a.

34 Martin Buber, *Tales of the Hasidim*, trans. Olga Marx (New York: Schocken Books, 1991), 251.

35 Reuben Zak, *Sefer Keneset Yisrael* (Warsaw 5666 [1905 or 1906]), 23.

36 The article Matemáticas subversivas (Subversive Mathematics), https://www.nexos.com.mx/?p=3404, was written by Mauricio Schoijet Glembotzky and published in Nexos (a Mexican magazine about politics, economy, society, science, art, and culture, founded in 1978 by the historian Enrique Florescano), on August 1, 1979. It deals with the prohibitions to teach certain scientific subjects, decreed by the military governments that were in power in Argentina between 1976 and 1983.

37 The King James Version also follows the Masoretic text in this instance and reads: "And Kayin talked with Hevel his brother; and it came to pass, when they were in the sadeh, that Kayin rose up against Hevel his brother, and killed him."

38 Genesis 4:17, 25; 1 Samuel 1:19; etc.

39 *Sifra' K'doshim, parashah* 2, *perek* 4, 12.

40 Matthew 22:36-40, Mark 12:28-33, Luke 10:25-29.

41   Pope Francis, *Fratelli Tutti*, 54. Available at https://www.vatican.va/content/
      francesco/en/encyclicals/documents/papa-francesco_20201003_enciclica-
      fratelli-tutti.html.

42   Ibid., 137.

43   See, for example, Deuteronomy 29:22, 32:32; Isaiah 1:9, 3:9; Jeremiah
      23:14; Amos 4:11; Lamentations 4:6; Zephaniah 2:9.

44   *b. Sanhedrin* 109a.

45   *b. Chullin* 91b; see Rashi's exegesis on *shehitpalelu vo avotai.*

46   *B'reishit Rabbah, parashat Vayishlach, parashah 77, siman* 3.

47   Excerpt from the *Advertencia* with which begins *Uno y el Universo* de
      Ernesto Sábato Universo, Seix Barral, Edición Definitiva, Buenos Aires,
      1996.

48   *b. Sanhedrin* 65b.

49   *The Hermeneutic and Alchemical Writings of Aureolus Philippus
      Theophrastus Bombast of Hohenheim, called Paracelsus the Great,*
      edited by Arthur Edward Waite, James Elliot and Co., London 1894,
      Vol. 1, p. 124.

50   Translation according to Ibn Ezra's exegesis.

51   *b. Sanhedrin* 65b.

52   *b. Shabbat* 97a.

53   Ibid.

54   *Leviticus Rabbah* (Vilna) 16:6.

55   *Leviticus Rabbah* (Vilna) 17:3.

56   *b. Berakhot* 35a-b.

57   *Midrash Rabbah, Emor, parashah* 31, *siman* 7.

58   Exegesis of Rashi on Numbers 8:2.

59   *b. Menachot* 86b.

60   *Yad Hachazakah, Hilchot Beit Hamikdash* 9:7, and Rabad's commentary
      ad locum.

61   *D'varim Rabbah* (Vilna), Ree, 4:4. Shimon bar Kappara' belonged to the
      first generation of *amora'im* from Israel.

62   *b. Shabbat* 31a.

63   For example, 1QS 9.10-11. See James H. Charlesworth, ed., *Rule of
      the Community and Related Documents, Vol 1: The Dead Sea Scrolls:
      Hebrew, Aramaic, and Greek Texts with English Translations* (Louisville:
      Westminster John Knox Press, 1994), 41.

64   4Q521. See Dr. James Tabor, "The Signs of the Messiah: 4Q521,"
      Archaeology and the Dead Sea Scrolls, University of North Carolina.
      Retrieved May 27, 2021. Available at https://pages.uncc.edu/james-
      tabor/archaeology-and-the-dead-sea-scrolls/the-signs-of-the-messiah-
      4q521/.

65   *b. Sanhedrin* 98b.

66   *b. Shabbat* 10a, 119b.

67   *b. Kiddushin* 68b.

68   *b. Shabbat* 118b.

69   *b. Yevamot* 61b.

70   *b. Yevamot* 63a.

71   *b.Yevamot* 62b.

72   1 Samuel 26:24, 2 Samuel 4:9, 2 Kings 19:3, Psalms 20:2, etc.

73   "Hadusi'ach bein Elohim Le'adam Bamikra, in *Te'uda ViY'eud*, ed. Hasifriyah HaTzi'onit (Jerusalem, 1959). There seems to be no English translation available of this article by Buber. This translation is my own.

74   *b. Bava Batra* 60b.

75   *Eichah Rabbah* 1.

76   *On Heaven and Earth*, 6-7.

77   *m. Shevi'it* 5:9, *m. Gittin* 5:8, etc., then *b. Gittin* 59b.

78   Dan Laor, *Hayye Agnon* (Tel Aviv: Schocken, 1998), 348-349.

79   *Si'ach Sarfei Kodesh*, vol. 1 (Lodz: 1932), 50, *siman* 233. Simcha Bunim Bonhardt of Peshischa (1765-1827), also known as the Rebbe Reb Bunim, was the second r of Peshischa (Przysucha, Poland) as well as one of the most prominent leaders of Chasidic Judaism in Poland.

80   *Midrash Elleh Ezkerah*, ed. Adolph Jellinek (Leipzig: 1853), 15; *Otzar Midrashim*, ed. Julius Eisenstein (New York: 1915), 443.

81   *b. Gittin* 56a-b.

82   The hope of rebuilding the Temple during the Tannaitic period is reflected in the Mishnah, *Ta'anit* 4:8 and *Tamid* 7:3; and in the *Tosefta*, *Rosh Hashanah* 2:9 (Lieberman); and in other places in the Babylonian and Jerusalem Talmuds. This hope is expressed in both daily and festival prayers.

83   "Poems," by Hannah Szenes, *The Jewish Week*, New York, December 22, 2010.